# YOGA
## BEYOND
## BELIEF

Insights to
Awaken and Deepen
Your Practice

GANGA WHITE

FOREWORD BY STING

North Atlantic Books
Berkeley, California

Published by
North Atlantic Books
P.O. Box 12327
Berkeley, California 94712

Cover and book design by
Suzanne Albertson
Printed in the United States of America

Unless otherwise noted, all photos are from Ganga White's archive collection.

Yoga Beyond Belief: Insights to Awaken and Deepen Your Practice is sponsored by the Society for the Study of Native Arts and Sciences, a nonprofit educational corporation whose goals are to develop an educational and crosscultural perspective linking various scientific, social, and artistic fields; to nurture a holistic view of arts, sciences, humanities, and healing; and to publish and distribute literature on the relationship of mind, body, and nature.

---

North Atlantic Books' publications are available through most bookstores. For further information, call 800-733-3000 or visit our website at www.northatlanticbooks.com.

---

Library of Congress Cataloging-in-Publication Data

White, Ganga.
    Yoga beyond belief: insights to awaken and deepen your practice / by Ganga White ; foreword by Sting.
        p. cm.
    Summary: "An integrative, new vision and context for yoga, illuminating its internal dynamics, providing inspiration and guidance for a lifetime of practice, and appealing to anyone practicing this tradition—from beginner to experienced student—this book offers a coherent explication of yoga's philosophy and practice"—Provided by publisher.
    Includes index.
    ISBN-13: 978-1-55643-646-8
    ISBN-10: 1-55643-646-7
    1. Hatha yoga. I. Title.
    RA781.7.W493 2007
    613.7'046—dc22                                                    2006024363
                                                                              CIP

    4   5   6   7   8   9   10   11   12   UNITED   14   13   12   11   10   09

*Dedicated to the development
of the total human being*

# ACKNOWLEDGMENTS

First, I would like to acknowledge the teachers and lineages who have handed down and expanded yoga through the ages. I especially acknowledge those who have given themselves the freedom and liberty to question, to test the boundaries, and to grow beyond the limitations of tradition into new expressions and new revelations. I honor my many teachers and many friends who have taught me what yoga is and, equally important, what it is not.

Thanks and appreciation go to my friend and compatriot, Mark Schlenz, for his editing wizardry. Great appreciation to Frank Rothschild and Evelyn de Buhr for their help, encouragement, and insight, and to Diana Alstad and Joel Kramer for many wonderful hours and long nights in the shared joy of inquiry.

Special thanks and appreciation go to Sting, David Gordon White, PhD, Jason Saleeby, PhD, Brent Derry, PhD, Joel Gotler, Jane Freeburg, Venkatesa—the laughing swami, J. Krishnamurti, all the editors and staff at North Atlantic Books, the staff of the White Lotus Foundation and Retreat in Santa Barbara, and so many others along the way.

And finally, with immeasurable gratitude, none of this would be possible without the love, support, joy, and partnership of the sublime, graceful, beautiful, and brilliant yogini, Tracey Rich.

# What if . . .

What if our religion was each other
If our practice was our life
If prayer, our words

What if the temple was the earth
If forests were our church
If holy water—the rivers, lakes, and oceans

What if meditation was our relationships
If the Teacher was life
If wisdom was self-knowledge
If love was the center of our being.

GANGA WHITE, for the Rainforest Benefit,
New York City, April 1998

# CONTENTS

FOREWORD The Yogi and the Shower Singer, by STING    xiii

INTRODUCTION Awakening Insight—Ganga White's
Approach to Yoga, by Mark Schlenz, PhD    xvii

CHAPTER ONE Standing On the Shoulders of the Past    I

Tradition and Interpretation    4

Freedom from the Known    7

A Fresh Point of View    8

CHAPTER TWO The Many Yogas    13

Raja, Hatha, and Tantra Yoga    16

Bhakti Yoga    18

Jnana Yoga    19

Karma Yoga    20

The Wholeness of Yoga    21

CHAPTER THREE Hatha—The Yoga of Sun and Moon    23

The Origins of Hatha Yoga    28

The Ten Body-Mind Systems    30

CHAPTER FOUR Finding the Ah Ha! in Hatha—
Principles, Hints, and Insights into Yoga Practice    37

Presence: Start Where You Are    39

The Long View    42

The Asanas Are Tools, Not Goals    43

Feedback: Learning to Listen    46

Strength and Flexibility    48

Heating and Cooling                                          50
The Rhythms and Seasons of Practice                          53
Tension Is Your Friend                                       54
Inner- and Outer-Directed Practices                          55
Mental Limitations                                           56
Fear As a Limitation                                         57
Competition and Comparison                                   58
Yoga Is for Every Body                                       59
There Is No Such Thing as Perfection                         61
Discipline                                                   62
Concentration and Attention                                  64
Using the Breath                                             65
The Ujjayi Breath                                            66
Toning the Spine                                             68
Symmetry and Alignment                                       69
The Three Qualities                                          71
The Three Root Principles                                    72
Relaxation                                                   73
Flow and Grace                                               74
Personal Practice                                            75
Integrating Yoga into Daily Life                             77
Enjoying Your Practice                                       80

CHAPTER FIVE  The Internal Alchemy of Hatha Yoga             81
The Dance of Energy                                          84
Aligning and Adjusting Asanas from Within and Without        91
Surfing the Edges                                            95
Flow, the Dance of Control and Surrender                     97
Pranayama—The Mastery of Energy                              99
Using Locks, or Bandhas                                     103
Traction, Torque, and Leverage                             105

The Nature of Balance 108

Advancing in Yoga 109

CHAPTER SIX Useful Styles and Modes of Practice 111

Flow Yoga 114

Intuitive Flow Yoga 116

Structural Integrity and Structural Archetypes 118

Active and Passive Holding 119

Long Holding 121

Odd-Day Practice 122

Car Yoga 122

The Neck and Lumbar 123

The Psoas, Quadriceps, and Hamstrings 124

Seven Classes of Asana 126

CHAPTER SEVEN Injury, Pain, and Healing 133

Pain Is Your Friend 137

There Is No Such Thing as Pain 140

Local Intelligence 141

Sympathetic Resonance 145

Causes and Prevention of Injury 146

Working with Injuries 148

CHAPTER EIGHT Chakras—The Play of Matter
and Energy 151

The Chakras' Relation to Science 155

Seven Energy Centers 156

Chakras and Levels of Being 159

The Cosmic Polarity 162

Chakras and Daily Life 164

CHAPTER NINE  Meditation Is Your Life                    167

    What Is Meditation?                                   169
    Can Meditation Be Practiced?                         171
    (There Is No) How to Meditate                        174
    Useful Meditation Practices                          177
    How Much to Practice                                 194

CHAPTER TEN  Spirituality, Enlightenment,
and the Miraculous                                      197

    Our Relation to the One                              200
    Oneness and the Loss of Diversity                    201
    Spirituality Beyond Belief                           202
    Evolutionary Enlightenment                           208
    The Mystery: Death and Time                          211
    Navigating Life                                      214

ABOUT THE AUTHOR                                        217

NOTES                                                   227

INDEX                                                   228

# FOREWORD

## The Yogi and the Shower Singer
### by STING

It may surprise you to read that someone who sings for a living like I do would enjoy singing in the shower as much as anybody else.

My shower, I suppose like most, has the kind of hard surface that reflects the notes back at you with a satisfying and friendly echo, almost as effectively as the walls of a church or an underground cavern or even the electronic reverb in a professional studio.

Admittedly, I don't sing what anyone would recognize as songs per se, nor do I use the shower fitting as a fantasy microphone, but instead limit myself to vocalizing long resonant tones. I will sustain a single OM for as long as my lungs can hold out, and advance semitone by semitone of the chromatic scale, beginning near the bottom of my range and gradually rising high enough for the sound to disturb the Labradors sleeping in the kitchen below. When they start to howl in sympathy (or agony, I can't tell which), I know it's time to dry off, shave, brush my teeth, clothe myself, and start the day.

As I enter the kitchen, the youngest of my six children greet me ironically, seated cross-legged at the breakfast table, chanting their own tuneless but grand, guttural OMs, eyes crossed and little hands flipping the bird in irreverent imitation of those mudras they've watched me assume at the end of my yoga practice.

"Good morning, my little philistines!"

"OHMMMMMMM ohmmmmmmmm ohmmmmmmmmm!"

"Why do you make that noise, daddy?"

Noise? Noise? I feign professional outrage while reaching for the coffee, black and bitter. Well, I suppose it's a fair question. Why *do* I make these noises? And why do I spend a good deal of my morning attempting to turn my body into a pretzel, while breathing like a telephone stalker, or chanting ancient unintelligible sounds in the echo chamber of my bathroom?

When my good friend Ganga requested that I write a foreword for his new book on yoga, I was both flattered and daunted by the task. While I've been practicing for more than fifteen years now, what do I really know about yoga? And has my fifteen years of practice changed me to any significant degree?

In fact, I don't spend a lot of intellectual energy thinking about yoga, or trying to articulate the processes it awakens, because, for one, I don't have to teach it, and, two, it's become an intrinsic part of my whole life, permeating it to such an extent that I don't really know where it begins or ends.

I have benefited from the wisdom of many teachers whose example has inspired me to undertake a voyage of discovery as complex and fascinating as music, through a realm that is mysterious, unexpected, and startling.

I have made a space for myself and my yoga practice every morning for fifteen years. I can perform feats of flexibility with my fifty-five-year-old body that I couldn't do when I was an athlete. That never ceases to amaze me, but is it the point?

"Part of yoga practice," Ganga has often reminded me, "is to connect."

And he makes his point clear: To connect flexibility and strength, balance, concentration, sexuality, consciousness, and spirituality, so that what may have begun solely as a physical practice can evolve into an integrated and holistic approach to all aspects of one's life.

For example, after Ganga's advice, my chosen profession of singing has morphed into yoga and yoga into singing.

Getting back to my shower practice, I will choose a low resonant tone and after a little practice I have learned to become aware not of this note I have chosen, but the subtle and ghostly harmonic five semitones above—the "dominant," as it is known. This note appears almost miraculously whenever you give it some attention. With a little more practice, further and yet higher resonances from the overtone scale reveal themselves, all related mathematically to the "tonic," my original note. Physics and metaphysics begin to blur here, as harmonic resonances beyond our hearing connect us to other realms.

Nada Brahma . . . the world is sound, so the sutras say.

Whatever seems solid and impermeable in this world is, at the molecular level, vibrating at pitches way beyond our range of perception. And this is the ultimate connecting principle.

My shower singing connects me at a molecular level to everything around me, to the frequency of the earth, and indeed with a leap of the imagination, to the cosmos or realms of dark matter.

And yoga, as my dear friend says, is to connect.

I've come to think of the asanas this way too—each position changing the frequency with which our bodies vibrate. To be conscious of this, as we breathe, turns the physical practice into a devotional one, connecting us via resonant vibration to the cosmos, tuning the instruments of our bodies to a higher "symphonic" purpose. A well-tuned instrument is a healthy instrument; yoga helps us resonate more efficiently with the universe.

I've also come to believe that the highest form of prayer is to pray and yet ask for nothing,

To resonate with awareness, acceptance, and gratitude is surely to pray,

To breathe and accept gratefully the air that surrounds me into my body.

Why a new yoga book? The world is chock full of orthodoxies—religious, pseudo-religious, political. These orthodoxies tend to assume that mankind is a finished product, that the "sacred" word is the final word. Such absolutism means that most of these true believers are unhappy with the idea of evolution, and some actively work to suppress it. *Yoga Beyond Belief* steps out of that limited mold. It will strike a chord with people seeking a new level of awakening and freedom in yoga and in their life. This book offers a flexible and modern perspective that is needed more than ever to live in these times of accelerating change.

Yoga has been pivotal and transformational in every aspect of my life. I regard myself as a work in progress. Yoga to me is an evolutionary, and indeed evolving, science, and orthodoxy needs to be challenged wherever it plants itself like a roadblock to progress. Of course, what is worth keeping will survive and continue to nourish future generations; whatever is moot and expendable will be proven so.

I am confident that Ganga's contemporary vision of yoga and the many tools he shares will be catalysts to aid readers in cultivating personal transformation. By combining ancient disciplines with cutting-edge knowledge and insights, this book can make yoga a living part of growth and development for those who practice any level of yoga and who have an interest in how yoga can be pertinent to modern living.

Ganga's lifelong study of yoga has not ossified into rigid modes of belief; indeed, his thinking is as flexible and improvisatory as his practice. His discipline is matched by his iconoclasm, his respect for the past by his courage to question authority in elucidating a new vision of yoga. Our human species' need to evolve has never been more critical. Yoga is one of the tools that can help us make that evolutionary leap and I believe this challenging book can help us redefine who we are and where we are going.

# INTRODUCTION

## Awakening Insight—
## Ganga White's Approach to Yoga

by Mark Schlenz, PhD

Ganga White has led the evolution of yoga in America for nearly four decades. He helped host yoga's arrival in this country during the sixties and seventies. He nurtured its development through the remainder of the twentieth century. Today, he remains at the forefront of yoga's ongoing transformation into the twenty-first century.

Once an officer in the Sivananda organization, Ganga established the first yoga centers in Los Angeles and several other major American cities. In 1968, his newly created White Lotus Foundation offered one of the first in-depth yoga teacher training programs in this country and established the working model for numerous programs that have since proliferated. Ganga's departure from Sivananda stimulated a major transformation in yoga's growth. Disillusioned by financial and ethical scandals involving the swamis, Ganga broke ties with traditional hierarchies of India, led the White Lotus to independence, and rededicated the foundation "to the development of the total human being" and to "elucidating a free, open, and contemporary approach to yoga." Since then, thousands of yogis now teaching in the United States and around the world have trained with Ganga at White Lotus and share his liberating perspectives with thousands more of their students.

As a leader of yoga's modern development, Ganga has always been nourished, rather than bound, by the past. Today, yoga's current popularity has given rise to a myriad of new market-driven forms and newly minted yogis. Much of what is currently marketed seems completely cut off from the vast richness of yoga's deep history. Yoga's age-old potential for fundamental transformation of the whole person is too often diluted to appeal to fashionable desires for physical attainments. Ganga's scholarly study and thorough immersion in the literature, philosophy, and techniques of ancient yoga traditions inform and inspire the evolution of his own dedicated practice and teaching. With this deep grounding, Ganga's innovative contributions build upon the vital essences of yoga's timeless gifts without subservience to archaic institutions or doctrines.

While many current yoga trends seem to disregard historical contexts, others tend to romanticize the past, fetishizing certain practices and depriving them of relevance to our current situations. Ganga's deeper understanding of yoga's many traditions recognizes how various practices emerged from specific historical, cultural, and social conditions and, even more important, how they have been consistently adapted as these conditions have inevitably changed through time. This dynamic sense of history nourishes Ganga's efforts to make yoga more relevant to our present *and* to our future. Through all its manifestations, yoga has always offered liberatory alternatives to rigid hierarchies that threaten the survival of the human spirit. At this moment, that spirit, and in fact all life on the planet, is more threatened than ever before. Our present potential for global annihilation, whether by our explosive weapons of mass destruction or by our escalating devastation of our own ecosystem, requires new orientations to preserve the human spirit's potential for creativity, healing, and love.

Incorporating essential wisdom from yoga's heritage with progressive insights of science and modernity, Ganga's evolutionary approach makes yoga more applicable than ever to addressing the overwhelming problems that currently confront every person. The crux of his insight is that we can certainly change the future of our species by constantly developing the ways we perceive and value our individual selves. Through constant self-examination and ongoing reflection, one's personal yoga practice becomes an invaluable tool for continual self-discovery and transformation.

Ganga's insights into dynamic principles animating the asanas enable his students to approach the poses as unfolding paths to personal evolution rather than as cul-de-sacs of arrested perfection. His teachings empower his students and allow them to let their own experiences guide them into deeper possibilities of personal growth and freedom. That is why this book, in contrast to so many yoga books written to formulas and dictates of the publishing market, offers principles rather than prescriptions.

Most yoga books currently published exploit niche market appeal by prescribing specific practices that promise certain benefits to particular audiences. Many claim the ancient authenticity of a particular tradition or lineage of teacher for their authority. Others rely on charismatic teachers or celebrities to underwrite their inflated promises. A growing number of hybrid approaches claim benefits only possible through newly created combinations of yoga with something—almost anything, it seems—else. *Yoga Beyond Belief* presents a unique, nondogmatic, integrative vision of contemporary yoga. It is an inspiring manual for beginners and experienced students alike.

What most available books share in common is the premise that they can give you something special by *telling you how to do yoga their way.* In this book, by contrast, Ganga *shows you how you can learn to do yoga your way.* What Ganga shares in the following chapters is not based on passed-down authority, fashionable popularity, or eclectic gimmickry. It is based on working principles of careful inquiry, experimentation, and observation.

Those of us who have had the fortune to learn from Ganga have learned much from watching his characteristic responses to questions from students. Perhaps an alignment he suggests contradicts an instruction a student has been taught by another teacher or has read some where, and so the student asks which is the right way. Older students who may have heard this question posed and answered more than once before know not to expect a definitive, or even the same, answer from Ganga.

What we know to expect instead is a demonstration of sincere inquiry, often enlivened with his spontaneous wit and infectious laughter. Almost invariably Ganga will experiment in the pose with the juxtaposed alignments before commenting on their relative merits and limitations as they might apply to different bodies, physical conditions, or stages of learning. Despite the newly discovered insights he might share in any instance, the consistency of his response is that it is definitely based in his immediate investigation as it builds upon his lifelong experience. Attentive students learn that this process, not the particular answer to any particular question, is the lesson.

That lesson is generously and repeatedly shared, along with splashes of Ganga's wit and stories, throughout this synthesis of his life's work. After providing a holistic overview of yoga traditions, *Yoga Beyond Belief* shares a wide range of functional principles, practical skills, and realistic attitudes that will empower you to evolve your own yoga practice. It encourages processes of self-discovery that will truly free and deepen your practice and your life and, so, enrich our world.

The introductory chapter, "Standing On the Shoulders of the Past," inspires an evolutionary perspective for contemporary yoga practitioners. This perspective is strengthened in the next chapters of the book through a comprehensive survey of various yoga forms in "The Many Yogas" and through a detailed analysis of the origins, history, and psycho-physical-spiritual principles in "Hatha—The Yoga of Sun and Moon."

In the book's central chapters, the practical insights of an evolutionary perspective are applied to specific aspects of Hatha yoga practice. "Finding the Ah Ha! in Hatha—Principles, Hints, and Insights into Yoga Practice" deals directly with many of the overarching questions, internal techniques, and attitudes yogis grapple with in developing a sustaining and dynamic personal practice. A practical context for pursuing a lifetime yoga practice is strengthened with more applications of concrete insights and experiential observations in "The Internal Alchemy of Hatha Yoga" and in "Useful Styles and Modes of Practice." Together, the contents, experiments, instructions, recommendations, and insights offered in these central chapters can liberate yoga students to learn from their own yoga practice and become their own yoga teachers. Practical considerations become particularly focused in "Injury, Pain, and Healing," where insights for healing and for learning from injury are offered from the author's experience.

The last group of chapters returns to a deeper exploration of philosophical contexts of yoga traditions in relation to contemporary practice. Yogic mappings of the subtle body are considered from an evolutionary perspective in "The Chakras—The Play of Matter and Energy." Then the nature of daily life itself is explored as a personal path of unfolding enlightenment in "Meditation Is Your Life"; in this chapter he shows that the real essence of meditation is free from obligatory, routine practices and techniques. Finally, "Spirituality, Enlightenment, and the Miraculous" reconnects the practical with the philosophical and rejoins the personal with the planetary as the evolutionary potential of the human spirit is reoriented to a liberating navigation of inquiry and insight. This final chapter challenges established definitions of enlightenment and presents a new, accessible vision of spirituality for modern times.

Attentive readers will learn how to apply insights offered here to their own experiences. Yoga students of all levels, from beginner to teacher, will learn to form and answer questions about their own practice through their own inquiry. As a result, this book offers yogis the most important benefits of yoga. *Yoga Beyond Belief* offers approaches to yoga that open possibilities for deep and liberating transformations of the self. It can certainly help guide all readers to an awakening of insight, free of archaic dependencies and romantic beliefs, and ready to meet the accelerating challenges of the twenty-first century.

*Dr. Mark Schlenz is a professor of creative writing and environmental studies at UC-Santa Barbara and a certified yoga teacher.*

# CHAPTER ONE

# Standing On the Shoulders of the Past

If I have seen further it is by standing on
the shoulders of giants.

—SIR ISAAC NEWTON, in a letter, circa 1676

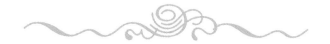

Yoga's growing popularity in the West raises many questions. For example, is yoga becoming "Americanized" and does that Americanization degenerate the purity or authenticity of the teachings? If yoga is being changed in the West, what right do we have to make these modifications? These concerns also raise deeper questions: What is the nature of tradition and authority? Can we truly know exactly what was taught and practiced in the past? Is there any actuality to the concept of "pure teachings" from the past?

I first realized the importance of these questions at a lecture series in the early seventies on one of the foundation texts of yoga, *The Yoga Sutras of Patanjali*. The lecturer was my great friend and mentor, Swami Venkates (1921–1982), a much-loved and respected yogi and Sanskrit scholar from India.[1] He explained that very little is actually known with much certainty about Patanjali, whom many consider one of the early codifiers, if not the father, of yoga. I use Patanjali as an example because his yoga sutras are used by many teachers as the touchstone of yoga, yet the text can be interpreted in widely differing manners. My swami friend emphasized that any translation or commentary on any text always involves someone's point of view. In fact, the translation process itself is interpretation. Even if we read or listen to a text in its original language, we must acknowledge that a large amount of personal interpretation still goes on in the way we receive it.

Language usage, meaning, and circumstance change over time. We have heard the story in Psychology 101 of the man who runs menacingly into and out of a classroom with a banana and the students are asked to write a report. Nearly everyone describes having witnessed the man doing different things; some saw the banana as a gun, a flashlight, or a telephone. What does this case of multiple interpretations of a single event imply about the possible purity of subtle teachings handed down over thousands of years? What should we learn about the limits of tradition and authority from our observation of the phenomenon of every major religion and tradition breaking down into dozens of sects and subgroups with conflicting opinions, often with each one asserting that only its members have the actual truth? Even secular laws written in contemporary times with clear intent are prone to conflicting interpretations. Carefully written laws can be stretched, interpreted, and argued in different directions. Spiritual concepts and teachings, especially from the ancient past, are far more vulnerable. Spirituality is not an exact science to be laid out in narrowly defined paths.

## Tradition and Interpretation

An adept scholar can find many different, often contradictory, meanings in the ancient texts. There are many examples in every tradition where, in order to support various philosophical positions, the same texts are translated in different ways. For example, some teachers believe Patanjali was an advocate, if not one of the originators, of Hatha yoga, while others assert that Patanjali's sutras do not support the practice of physical yoga at all. When I first started teaching, I mentioned in a class that I was taught that the sutras were the foundation of Hatha yoga. A few days later a well-known elder swami from another organization called me and angrily chastised me, asserting that Patanjali was not at all an advocate of physical yoga. He stated that Patanjali's mention of *asana* and *pranayama,* posture and breathing, only referred to sitting quietly and stilling the breath for meditation. The swami said spending time and energy to cultivate the body would lead to attachment, body consciousness, and would detract one from the true spiritual path. This opinion is the antithesis of what most modern, Western yoga students believe.

Another example of differing opinions in the yoga sutras is the word *brahmacharya.* Usually translated as celibacy and abstinence, brahmacharya has also been reinterpreted by some teachers in modern times to mean responsible sexuality or spiritual sexuality aimed toward God. This shows how the same text can be assumed to have opposite meanings. There are texts that prescribe renunciation in order to attain godhood and those that say indulgence is the path. Some ancient scriptures say the doors of heaven are only open to vegetarians and others that say the opposite. I remember Swami Venkates pointing out that yogic texts and teachings are so vast and so complex that we can find traditional support and authority for almost anything we want to do. In spite of these limitations, students and teachers often spend great energy in debate to try to bolster an edict or find an exact meaning of a Sanskrit sutra in English. This quest may ever elude them. How can truth or the immensity of life and spirit be confined and captured in explanation? How can wisdom and spiritual realization be attained by mechanical processes or the practice of specific techniques? In this book you will see how these questions or problems should not cause us despair but, rather, strengthen us in following our hearts and minds.

Yoga is a cherished and valuable tradition. We can learn from and use the tradition in an approach tempered by the realization that what we call tradition is truly our own, or another's, interpretation of what something *may have been* in the distant past. My swami friend Venkates suggested that we use ancient writings to stimulate our inquiry and to catalyze our direct perception and understanding of our own lives without becoming overly dependent on tradition. Relying too much on doctrines and texts for guidance in living cuts one off from direct perception and from the living awareness of insight. Yoga should be viewed as an art as well as a science. Structured, more scientific, aspects of yoga and techniques also involve unstructured, indefinable dynamics that require artistry and awareness to apply. Living in wholeness and creativity has structural components, but life is more an art than a science. Even in asana practice there is structure as well as the artistry of application to the individuality of the person and the moment. Yoga is practiced within the tradition but must be applied according to the uniqueness of each person's life and situation. We should not simply idealize the past and assume that teachings, purportedly unchanged from the ancient past, are perfect, superior, or appropriate for the present. It is impossible truly to know the ancient past. Giving teachers, and even teachings, the status of perfection is the beginning of authoritarianism and a recipe for abuse. When teachers say they are presenting a perfected teaching, there is the veiled implication of unquestionable authority. The teacher is elevated as the pure vessel of this perfected path. It is important to be aware of what power, stature, and position a particular viewpoint gives to the teacher expounding it. There is no single interpretation of yoga. We cannot learn to fly by following the tracks left by birds in the sand. We must find our own wings and soar.

Another great teacher, J. Krishnamurti, said, "The observer is the observed," meaning, among other implications, that when we study something it is affected and colored by our own interpretations and projections. This influence is also a problem in setting up scientific experiments. The way the experiment is set up affects the outcome. Is light matter or energy? It turns out that it depends on how we look at it. The method of observation has a direct relationship to the way the observed object is perceived. Krishnamurti also said, "Truth has no path, and that is the beauty of truth, it is living. A dead thing has a path to it because it is static."[2] He pointed out that because we have exactness and authority in the technological world, we unconsciously carry the ideas of authority and structure over to the spiritual arena where they have no place. We are living, changing beings. We can learn from and honor tradition and we can also grow beyond it to develop the ability to listen to our own uniqueness by incorporating contemporary insights and discoveries. If we are too busy trying to relive the past, we may miss birthing the new. We do not have to limit ourselves to searching backwards through the musty corridors of the ancient past for answers to the mutating and constantly changing questions of the living present. Tradition can be valuable and useful, but we should not forego the much more relevant insights that can be found right here and now on our own yoga mats, and in the laboratory of our own lives.

## Freedom from the Known

An insatiable appetite and energy for learning and a fresh inquiring mind are among life's greatest assets. This is why the concept of *beginner's mind* has been emphasized in the East. When we come to learning as a beginner, we are open, questioning, looking. When we approach a subject as an expert, we are more closed and fixed in the accumulated information we have gathered, in the past experiences we have had. When we're an expert, or experienced, when we *know* something, even a yoga posture, we tend to approach it mechanically, from the past. We lose the freedom of discovery, the freedom of being fresh and new.

As our journey in the unending process of learning and growing in wisdom progresses, we must endeavor to keep a fresh context, a fresh attitude, a beginner's mind. We must keep the content we acquire from hardening and clouding the context in which we hold information and experience. Our context, the ground of being with which we hold the information, should be kept open, flexible, and free.

There is an ancient saying: "He who knows, knows not. And he who knows not, knows." Or: "He who knows doesn't say. And he who says, doesn't know." One of the messages of this saying is that there is much more to wisdom and understanding than mere knowledge and information. Knowledge and information are limited, as there is always room for growth and change. One who thinks he *knows* doesn't understand this limitation and has therefore a restricted perception. One who sees his or her own limitations, and the limits of knowledge, may actually see more clearly. The word *intelligence,* from *inter legere,* means to see between the lines. Intelligence is seeing between the hard lines of fixed information and knowledge, having the subtle, flexible perception that can see beyond the norm, beyond limited definition and formula. I once heard a very wise man discussing this concept and also what brings about a state of clear intelligence and penetrating perception. His inquiry revealed that the necessary ground for awakening intelligence is an open state of consciousness that begins with *not knowing.* Saying "I don't know" is the beginning of the awakening intelligence. As this wise man was explaining this, he looked up at his questioner and said, "And you don't know either!" pointing out that this type of seeing does not happen by looking to others to fill our void. The vulnerable state of humility, of saying "I really don't know" opens one to discovery—but we must also be vigilant not to allow ourselves to become susceptible to those who would like to fill us with their dogmas and doctrines.

## A Fresh Point of View

A famous Zen story is told about a student coming to learn from a wise teacher. During the introductions the student tries to show his worthiness to the teacher by narrating a history and explanation of his studies. The teacher begins to pour the student a cup of tea while listening to the monologue. He fills the cup, then keeps pouring until it overflows onto the table and into the student's lap, causing him to jump up and shout at the teacher, saying, "How could you! You're supposed to be an aware person; can't you see my cup is full?" The teacher replies, "Yes, your cup is full. You're so full of yourself, in fact, that there's no room for anything new. Please come back when your cup has some space in it." This story points out that we must have inner space and receptivity to learn. But I have never heard this popular parable looked at from the perspective of the student. Spiritual teachers are usually assumed to have authority and higher knowledge. The story can be seen to cut both ways, however, and can also point to the teacher being so full of himself and what he has to offer that he devalues the student's knowledge and chastises him.

The idea of keeping a fresh, open context and not getting stuck in explanations, words, and descriptions resonates in the first verse of the honored, ancient text, the *Tao Te Ching*. Verse one of the Tao says, "The Tao that is explained is not the Tao. Now an explanation of the Tao." With that opening paradox and contradiction, the teacher cautions that his explanation only points toward something—toward direct perception and revelation. We need to teach and educate each other, but we must be careful not to get stuck in the words we use to do so. We are cautioned in the beginning not to get stuck in the text, the words of the Tao that follow. Instead, we are urged to see beyond words, to see what the words are pointing toward.

In Sanskrit, a *mahavakya* refers to a great saying or formula that should be contemplated. *Tat Twam Asi,* meaning Thou Art That, is considered by many to be one of the greatest mahavakyas. We see in many ancient Sanskrit texts the word *Tat,* or That, used to point toward the sacred, the immeasurable. The English word *that* comes from the Sanskrit word Tat. It is interesting and informative to note that this great saying uses the word *that* instead of a description, a specific name, or a less abstract word. *That* is a word used to point. When we point our finger we often say "that." This word was chosen in this great saying to remind us it is pointing toward something we should not overly describe and limit with words and names. Overly describing, defining, or personifying the sacred leads to division and religious conflict. We are all part of the infinite, the immeasurable, the ineffable. *You are that.*

The word *Vedanta* also points toward freedom from the limitations of knowledge. Vedanta is one of the ancient yogic philosophical systems. The word *Veda* means knowledge and *anta* means *the end.* Vedanta is the end of the ancient Vedas and is often said to imply the end philosophy or the highest philosophy. The double entendre and hidden message in the word Vedanta is that it also means the *ending of knowledge,* or freedom from the known—that which is beyond the known. A central practice in Vedanta is negation—discovering the actual by removing, or negating, what it is not. For example, if you negate or remove arrogance, humility may come into being. There is a related form of inquiry or meditation approach called *Neti Neti*—not this, not this. Neti Neti aims one toward the realization that the transcendent cannot be contained in an object. We can explain love but love itself remains beyond words. By removing what is not love from our lives, we create more possibility for love to come into being. The greatest things in life are not obtained simply by acquiring knowledge of them.

As a final example to point out the distinction between context and content, between the accumulation of knowledge and that which is beyond, consider a modern koan. A *koan* is a cosmic riddle pondered to achieve an insight that catalyzes a nonrational flash of understanding and illumination. One of the most famous such koan questions is, "What is the sound of one hand clapping?" In koan style inquiry, one isn't supposed to circumvent the process by giving the answer. The process of questioning, pondering, and breaking the riddle yields a light of understanding.

A humorous, modern Zen koan addresses the paradox of contradiction encountered when trying to convey the teachings. In this story a teacher gives a student a question to solve: "How many Zen masters does it take to screw in a light bulb?" After working for weeks on the riddle, the student finally has a flash of seeing. "It takes two," he says. "One to screw the light bulb in and one *not* to screw it in!" The student saw that the true meaning of Zen lies in the explanations and at the same time is beyond them. Words and descriptions can only be part of the equation, part of the actual. That which lies between the lines cannot be conveyed in words.

This book raises many questions, perhaps more than it answers. It is often more important to question our answers than to answer our questions. The process of questioning and holding a question within ourselves becomes part of the light on the path of discovery, softening and opening us to new realizations. When we trust ourselves enough to begin to question tradition and authority, we begin the process of direct discovery. It has been said that the highest learning comes in four parts: One part is learned from teachers; another part from fellow students; a third part from self-study and practice; and the final part comes mysteriously, silently, in the due course of time. Inquiry and questioning can free us from the rigid, mechanical life of strict adherence to one belief, and can move us into the joy of continuous learning.

Once, while walking in the mountains, an old Chinese teacher said to me, "If I teach you, you must stand on my shoulders." This is a beautiful metaphor. We don't throw away tradition: we stand on the shoulders of the past to find how we can see a bit farther.

CHAPTER 2

# The Many Yogas

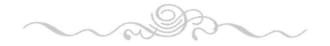

*i*t usually is not long after one begins study of yoga that a myriad of types of yoga are encountered. A few types are *Hatha, Jnana, Bhakti, Karma, Kundalini, Kriya, Atma, Agni, Buddhi, Parama, Tantra, Laya,* and *Mantra* yogas. These divisions can become quite confusing. The word *yoga* comes from the word *yuj,* which means to yoke, or connect. The English root, *jug,* as in *jug*ular or con*jug*ate, has the same origin. Yoga signifies *union,* to unite or make whole. How has this science of reintegration itself become divided into so many seemingly conflicting parts? In order to understand this we must first look at a few of the major systems.

Though there are many different lineages, or names, of yoga systems, modern yogis tend to categorize yoga into four or five major branches. These are sometimes referred to as The Four Yogas. When analyzing just about any approach, or brand, of yoga, one usually finds it is made up of components from the major four branches. I will offer here a simple introduction to the big four and some of the strengths and possible pitfalls of each. It is important to realize that modern interpretations of yoga, and Hatha yoga in particular, are actually syncretic amalgams taken from many ancient and contemporary beliefs and practices. Any definition of yoga is interpretive; the presentation here is limited to the basics of these yoga systems, with a new perspective on them.

## Raja, Hatha, and Tantra Yoga

*Raja* means king, and Raja yoga is known as the kingly yoga. This yoga is usually attributed to Patanjali, who first codified this system, although he did not call it Raja but simply a vision of yoga. It was actually Swami Vivekananda (1863–1902) who popularized and systemized this approach. Patanjali's teachings are found in a treatise consisting of four volumes of *sutras,* or brief aphorisms, which go into the analysis and explanation of psychology, mental states, the cause and removal of suffering and delusion, and psychic and magical powers. His two most-quoted sutras are *Yogas chitta vritti nirodaha* and *Yama, niyama, asana, pranayama, pratyahara, dharana, dhyana, samadhi.* These aphorisms are translated in various ways, often with subtle or profound differences in meaning. The first one, for example, is often translated as "Yoga is the stilling of mental turbulence" or "Yoga is the control of the mental modifications." The second sutra is a list of eight practices and might be translated as "Yoga consists of observances, abstinences, posture, control of life force, turning the senses inward, concentration, meditation, and super-consciousness or reintegration." Followers of Raja yoga usually see these as the eight limbs or steps of yoga and hence this system is also called *Ashtanga* yoga, or eight-limbed yoga. Hatha yoga is often included as part of Raja yoga, because of its second and third limbs, asana and pranayama, but Hatha almost certainly evolved several centuries later. Many practitioners also see Hatha yoga as a separate and complete system.

Although many modern proponents of Hatha yoga attribute its roots and foundations to Patanjali and to Raja yoga, Hatha's origins are actually more connected to a later form, Tantra yoga. Tantra differs from traditional yoga, which tends to center around ascetic and renunciative practices and beliefs, in that Tantra seeks spiritual development through the mundane. The Tantric path cultivates awakening in daily life through the feminine, goddess worship, sexuality, and even limited intoxication. Modern definitions of yoga, Hatha yoga, and Tantra are actually blended from many ancient and contemporary beliefs and practices.

Some forms of contemporary yoga and Tantra involve sexual practices and meditations. Sex can be one of the deepest and most profound meditations and influencers of consciousness. It is the meditation of birth and death with the potency of the wholeness of life. To deny sexuality is to deny the creative force of life. One could say a lot about Tantra, and the yoga of love, but modern Tantra can be distilled down to exploring how to discover and strengthen love, relationship, and connection, while riding the waves of creative force that is the dance of sexuality. Some yogic lineages suggest that it is necessary to limit or deny the sexual in order to be near what they call the purity of God. It may be possible to connect with God and Goddess spiritually through such renunciation and denial, but this far more often leads to repression and neurosis than it does to spiritual awakening. Denial, or attempted sublimation, is much more difficult than is riding the wave of all the senses, of sexuality, connection, love, and relationship. Raja yoga puts its emphasis on controlling ourselves while Tantra shows the importance of letting go to life and merging in the bliss of love.

One of the appealing things about Raja yoga is also its very limitation. It appears to be a scientific, step-by-step path to truth or enlightenment. This makes it especially attractive to the Western mind which seeks order and explanation for everything. It is the yoga of control, and what is more controlling than a king? Most interpretations of Raja yoga emphasize controlling the mind, the senses, the life force, thought, breath, and most other aspects of life. Control is a seductive concept because it mesmerizes us with the illusion that if we could only completely control ourselves, control our actions, do our practices properly, and follow the rules, we would live in harmony and attain the goal of life and highest wisdom. On the contrary, the more controlling we are, the more hardened, rigid, and out of tune with the flow of life we can become. We must learn the importance of control in our lives but also its limits. Control is necessary, but an excess limits us and we can become rigid and mechanical.

## Bhakti Yoga

Bhakti yoga is the yoga of devotion, consisting of prayer, singing, devotional practices, study of scriptures, remembrance of God, service, and rituals. It is the branch of yoga most similar to world religions. Bhakti yoga is based on cultivating faith and devotion and its goal is total surrender to God. It acknowledges that our own mind and understanding are limited, and therefore it behooves us to attune to and serve God, or, for the less theistic person, to serve and endeavor to live in tune with higher intelligence in the universe. Bhakti yoga seeks to lead us toward what is described as the bliss and ecstasy of oneness with God. It points out the limits of personal will, effort, and control, and the necessity of learning to surrender to the higher powers of life, death, and divinity. Bhakti suggests there is a limit to what we can attain by ourselves and purports that divine grace is necessary for spiritual development. Bhakti is the path of the heart, but followed blindly or to extremes can lead to the ignorance of ritualism, emotionalism, and mindlessness.

A modern approach to Bhakti yoga is directing devotion to the magic, mystery, and beauty of life and the operation of higher levels or orders of intelligence. Devotion can take many forms and is not limited to external prayers, chanting, and rituals. This understanding is not just a matter of belief. It is possible to go beyond the type of faith that is the belief in the promises of doctrines and the assertions of others. This deeper level is devotion to the movement of constant discovery and unveiling of deeper layers of meaning and order that opens the doors to new discoveries and to questioning the realizations of today, so the possibility remains of broadening and deepening awareness each moment. The devotional path instructs us to learn to live from our hearts, guided by love, faith, compassion, and the interconnectedness of all things.

## Jnana Yoga

Jnana yoga is the yoga of wisdom, based on the study of oneself and everything in life. This yoga suggests that we cannot merely cultivate the supreme qualities in life, such as divine love, truth, or God consciousness. These *non-things* cannot be brought into being by our limited minds and limited actions. Rather, they come into being when we remove the obstructions of our own ignorance and illusions. In its non-dualist forms, Jnana even denies that we are ever separate from God. It asserts that acts of worship or seeking of God in fact strengthen our separateness and deny the oneness that already exists. The famous saying Tat Twam Asi (Thou Art That) points to the fact that we are already at one with the sacred. As we have shown, this saying not only asserts oneness but carefully uses the word *that* to point to truth instead of naming or defining it. Rather than being based on faith, Jnana yoga encourages inquiry and questioning. In that sense it is very scientific. It is the yoga of seeing and being, asking us to question, look, and discover rather than to follow and believe. Faith is elevated in so many religious perspectives while questioning and doubt are limited or denigrated. Einstein said, "The important thing is never to stop questioning." Questioning and doubt are important allies that guide us and push and lead us to so many discoveries and insights.

Questioning does not imply a lack of faith and devotion. It is faith and devotion operating at a different level—the faith that comes into being through direct perception. A Jnana yogi sees the magic, mystery, and beauty of life and the operation of higher levels of intelligence. He or she aims to go beyond the faith that is the belief in the words and promises of doctrines and the assertions of others. A modern approach to Jnana and Bhakti yoga encourages devotion to more essential higher principles of life rather than to sectarian religious deities. In this time of intensifying religious wars, we must constantly endeavor to understand and deprogram our consciousness from ritualistic and sectarian beliefs, however old and cherished, that divide us and are the cause of so much killing and planetary degradation. We might better direct our devotion toward the great common denominators of higher perception, the great guiding principles of love, truth, common humanity, the sacredness of life and our planet, and the highest good of all. This is not just a secular, humanist point of view—it is the essence of spirituality.

Jnana yoga has been called the *pathless path*. It endeavors to free us from conditioning and the limitations of knowledge. It shows us that when we open our eyes and begin to see the beauty and sacredness around us we have less need of techniques, rituals, or beliefs. An ancient yogic text, *Bhagavad Gita,* says, "For one who has seen the infinite, all the sacred texts are of as much use as a container of water in a place where there has been a flood." We need to end our illusion and delusion. This happens through the awakening of perception and watchfulness in our daily life. But imbalanced practice of Jnana can lead to cynicism, excessive intellectualism, or dry, mental self-indulgence.

## Karma Yoga

Karma yoga is the yoga of action, the yoga of doing. We must live and act in the world, and this branch of yoga seeks to bring more awareness and artistry into our actions. It deals with both the quality and the motivation of action and could be called the *yoga of doing.* Karma yoga urges us to learn to act with clarity, wholeness, artistry, and meditation in action. Our businesses, our bodies, our relationships, and even how we do the dishes, with right understanding, all become expressions of our yogic awareness. Our actions are the manifestation of our inner reality. As is often said, we can talk the talk, but do we walk the walk?

Karma yoga is the place where all yoga systems can come together. No matter what our point of view, when spiritual awareness awakens and the heart opens with love and compassion, its expression is in sharing it with others. A danger of yoga, and of life itself, is excessive self-centeredness. Most yoga practices deal with improving our minds, bodies, and hearts so we must be vigilant about becoming preoccupied with ourselves. Yoga is something far deeper than developing the body beautiful or increasing personal bliss. Karma yoga also reminds us to think of and serve others, especially those who cannot help themselves— the poor, the sick, the elderly. Karma yoga asserts that "you are the world."

## The Wholeness of Yoga

To our unawakened eye these branches of yoga may seem to contradict each other. Bhakti says have faith, while Jnana says question everything. Raja says control your mind, while Jnana says the controller is that which you are trying to control. Bhakti says pray, serve, and surrender to God, while Jnana says prayer and ritual can strengthen separation— that we must see instead that we are already one with God. We may perceive the unity of these branches when we understand that yoga practices are tools to help us on our journey, rather than means or paths to an end or goal. When we have seen that there is no path to truth, that truth and spirit are living things, then the limbs of yoga can serve us as useful practices and guiding tools that we use on our journeys.

Perhaps the metaphor of a sage will help. He likened the four yoga branches to the parts of a bird. Raja yoga is the tail, steering, steadying, and guiding the bird with control. Karma is the yoga of action; it is the wings propelling the bird onward. Bhakti is the heart, guiding with love and compassion. And Jnana is the head, piloting the bird toward the light with perception and vision. Which part can we deny and still fly?

The four yogas actually point to four key qualities or capacities that balance each other—faith balanced by questioning or doubt, and control balanced by surrender or letting go. These qualities are essential polarities in our internal guidance systems. Any one of these can be out of balance, but used together they give different perspectives that guide us on our path.

CHAPTER 3

# Hatha—The Yoga of Sun and Moon

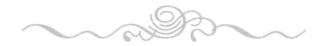

When most people think of yoga, they immediately think about the most popular form of yoga in the Western world today: Hatha yoga. Today, we find images of yogis and yoginis in every type of attire, situation, and exotic pose in nearly every popular media around the globe. Still, just as comparatively little is generally known about the other branches of the yoga tradition, the term "Hatha yoga" is often lost in a confusion of various *brand names* such as Power yoga, Fire yoga, Water yoga, Flow yoga, Ashtanga, and myriad other types of yoga named for or by influential teachers. All of these approaches, however, have common roots in Hatha yoga, the yoga of sun and moon. Made up of the syllables *Ha* meaning sun and *Tha* meaning moon, the word *Hatha* (pronounced ha tuh) actually means "intense" or "vigorous" and refers to the physical practices of yoga.

The reasons for the great popularity of this form are many. It has benefits that one can experience from the first practice and it may be the original system of holistic health dealing with all aspects of living. Hatha yoga is also endless—we can swim its seas as far or as deeply as our interest and energy carry us. The nuances and subtleties of discovery are boundless. There is no end to the potential of learning and no limit to the frontier, which is why it has been called a fount of perpetual wisdom. We will certainly pass through difficulties and pains, but there is so much enjoyment and benefit to the practice that it carries us throughout life.

While Hatha yoga refers to physical yoga, and it is certainly the branch with the most physical techniques and practices, it is not merely an exercise system. The very word Hatha implies a perspective of universal polarity and interplay of opposites. Remember, while the word Hatha actually means forceful, intense, or vigorous, Hatha creates awareness of subtle energies and the play of dynamic opposites. Hatha yoga is both a vast art and a science. It is a science because of its highly refined practices and techniques, and an art because the ever-changing nature of life cannot be limited merely to a definable system or mechanistic structure. Hatha yoga involves the physical practices of asana (yoga postures), pranayama (control of breath and energy), bandhas (muscular locks and contractions), mudras (seals and gestures), kriyas (internal cleansing techniques), philosophies, and meditations.

The word yoga in the West is nearly synonymous with Hatha yoga, but this is not so in India, its birthplace. There, yoga refers to a large array of spiritual philosophies and disciplines of which Hatha is just one part. Thousands of yogis and yoga lineages in India have no Hatha or asana practice at all. They focus on meditation, devotional, or philosophical practices. Some lineages actually denigrate physical practices. They believe that attention to the physical body detracts one from spiritual life and creates inappropriate attachment to the body. Hatha yogis deny this separation.

I once heard a story about an incident at a yoga congress in India. A Hatha yoga master just completed a demonstration and talk on the importance of caring for the body and the body's effects on mental and spiritual life. The organizer of the conference, hoping for some fireworks, had mischievously followed this speaker on the program with a swami who was known to disagree with Hatha practice. He represented a philosophical system that emphasized purely mental and inner practices.

The swami began his talk, in which he "humbly" pointed out that, as impressive as Hatha practices are, they actually create illusion and attachment to the body. He went on to assert that the body is just an aging sack of bones, blood, and hair that will die no matter what we do. (This description may sound grotesque, but it is not that uncommon to find the body referred to this way in ancient texts that promote renunciation and detachment from the physical.) The swami continued, getting heated up and raising his voice with authority declaring that when one attains spiritual insight he would pay no attention to the body whatsoever. At this moment the first speaker got up from his chair on the stage, slipped behind the swami, and removed the thick eyeglasses the swami was wearing! "Don't pay any attention to your body whatsoever, Swami! Detach, detach!" he shouted. "Maybe you shouldn't even eat or take medicine either. Where do you draw the line?" The debate went on, I'm told, until the nearly blind swami was forced to plead for the return of his glasses.

One of the beauties of Hatha yoga is that it acknowledges the interrelationship of body, mind, and spirit and explores the interactions and relationships along the body-mind continuum. Hatha yoga is predicated on the perception of a relationship between body, mind, and spirit and the appreciation of the journey of constant learning from the intelligent forces dwelling within all things. The laws of the external universe are also the laws of the internal universe. Hatha yogis see the physical and spiritual as reflecting and affecting each other, and as one process and interplay along one spectrum of energy. What happens within the body affects the mind, heart, and spirit—and the reverse is equally true. The divinity we see outside ourselves is part of the same sacred energy of life that is the body. The deeper levels of Hatha aim to bring this perception to the practitioner.

## The Origins of Hatha Yoga

Many beliefs and theories claim to explain the origins of Hatha yoga. They range from the scientific, based on archeological, anthropological, and etymological studies, to the folkloric, religious, and mythological. Scientists and scholars study and give credence only to actual historical proof to support their positions. Historical evidence has shown that the twelfth- and thirteenth-century teacher, Gorakhnath, was the original synthesizer of Hatha yoga and that, according to traditional lore, Matsyendranath (assumed to be of the tenth century) was Gorakhnath's guru, although there is no evidence for this belief.

Traditionalists, gurus, and believers rely on oral transmission, personal meditations, and the beliefs of their lineages. Yoga origin beliefs abound in India. Many Indian yogis assert that God or divine incarnations revealed or handed yoga down—it is a gift from the gods. Others suggest that great sages discovered yoga through meditation and divine communication or that they developed it through self-study and observation of animals. The exact origins of yoga may remain unknown and lost in antiquity. What is known is that these teachings have been preserved, expanded upon, and handed down through the ages from teacher to student because of their cherished value and benefits, as well as for the power thus assured for the teacher.

In Hindu mythology the domain of yoga, especially Hatha yoga, is often given to Siva, who is known as the destroyer in the Hindu trinity of gods that also includes Brahma, the creator, and Vishnu, the preserver. The concept of Siva as destroyer actually points toward the process of transformation because energy changes form—it is transformed, but is not destroyed. So Siva's destructive power can also be understood as a release of creative energy. In this role, then, Siva is the god of transformation, and because yoga is the art and science of transformation, Siva is also called the lord of yoga. Yoga seeks to transform the lower into the higher, ignorance to wisdom, and sickness to health.

There is a great origin myth for Hatha yoga. In one variation of this myth, Siva was visiting Earth with his wife or consort, Shakti. By the banks of a lake he decided to give her a demonstration of yoga asanas. It is said there are 840,000 different yoga postures and since Siva, the creator of this yoga, would certainly know them all, this performance must have taken a good bit of time. Shakti became bored after awhile with his long display and fell asleep. When Siva noticed her inattention he was angry that his fabulous spectacle was being wasted on his wife. Then he noticed that a fish was near the lake's surface intently watching everything. Siva thought, "This fish has better concentration and is more interested in yoga than my sleeping wife. I will make him a great yogi." The fish was turned into a man, called Matsyendranath, which means lord or king of the fish, and Matsyendranath became the first yogi. There may have historically been a man named Matsyendranath who lived during the tenth century and who actually was one of the earliest originators of Hatha yoga.

In much of modern belief and folklore, East and West, Hatha yoga is said to be thousands of years old. Scientific and academic research has found no validation for this claim. The broader philosophical and spiritual dimensions of yoga and other branches do go back millennia, but Hatha is probably much younger, originating around the first millennium CE (of the Common Era, or Christian Era). Modern folklore and many traditional yogis tend to idealize Hatha yoga's past and feel that very early on it was a highly perfected form of physical and spiritual development with practices for health, well-being, and mental clarity. On the contrary, academicians have asserted that the earliest forms of Hatha were oriented toward the attainment of supernatural and magical powers or physical immortality. The teachings and definition of Hatha yoga have grown and expanded enormously in modern times, incorporating many new discoveries and innovations, and integrating much from science. These changes and developments do not devalue the practice but, on the contrary, have strengthened and built it far beyond its humble origins. They further emphasize the evolutionary nature of yoga and the importance of constant questioning, vigilance, and feedback in the process.

## The Ten Body-Mind Systems

Hatha yoga, intelligently practiced, has extraordinary, beneficial effects on many levels, physically, mentally, and spiritually. As it has been handed down and expanded through the centuries, it has evolved, continually, into the most complete and sophisticated system of physical culture, health, and well-being ever known to humanity. Yoga practices work with and balance many interrelationships within body and mind. In order to have a more holistic understanding of how yoga works, ten body-mind systems can be taken into account. The spectrum of the ten systems, from the dense, physical bones of the skeletal system to amorphous consciousness of the mental system, is a holographic parallel to the matter-energy continuum of the physical universe and to the levels of energy of the chakra system, which we will explore in a later chapter. These ten systems are closely interrelated and their functions overlap. Getting a sense of the actions and relationships of these ten can be very useful in the practice and understanding of yoga.

### The Skeletal System

Our bones are the densest parts of our bodies. Though we might tend to think our skeletal system has grown and developed to a complete and static form and strength by the time we reach maturity, in fact our bones are living tissue that can be strengthened through use or weakened by inactivity throughout life. This dynamic fact was clearly evident to astronauts living in the weightless environment of space. Beyond Earth's pull of gravity, astronauts' bones begin to decalcify and their muscles weaken. As a result, systems of exercise that use springs and internal tensions are necessary in space travel and space stations are designed to revolve, simulating gravity with centrifugal force. The skeletal system is stimulated to strengthen and remain strong by the weight-bearing effects of yoga practice. Additionally, yogis learn how to move and mobilize all of the joints, where bone meets bone, in the body. A balanced practice has upper-body work and weight bearing on many body parts and moves and articulates all of the body's joints.

## The Muscular System

The skeletal structure is supported and articulated by the muscular system. A healthy, balanced muscular system requires more than just strong, toned muscles. To maintain the symmetry and alignment of the body, muscular tensions on different sides of the body and within opposing muscle sets are equalized by yoga practice. Excessive resistance and tension within the muscles waste energy. Muscles strengthened and lengthened by yoga are less prone to injury than short, tight muscles and they work and use energy more efficiently. Yoga asana practice teaches us how to use, tone, build, and balance the muscular system.

## The Circulatory System

Numerous medical studies have shown the important health benefits of building and maintaining good circulation in the cardiovascular system. Good circulation involves blood, lymph, and all the bodily fluids. Good health, vitality, and immunity require keeping fluids moving well in veins, arteries, capillaries, the lymphatic system, and even in the bones, marrow, and spinal disks. Pumping and working the circulatory system on a daily basis is key for health, well-being, detoxification, and the relief of tension. Asana practice has many unique circulatory effects. Many postures direct circulatory flows to specific body parts, glands, or organs. Using inversions like the Headstand, Shoulderstand, and even Downward Dog, for example, bring increased circulation to the upper body, the head, neck, face, and scalp, as well as the thyroid, pineal, and pituitary glands. The many compressing and squeezing actions in yoga postures assist the heart in keeping fluids moving, preventing stagnation. These circulatory benefits and effects also work on the lymphatic system fluids, which are vital to health and the immune system. Health experts have long pointed out that pumping and circulating one's bodily fluids through exercise is one of the most important factors in health and disease prevention.

The circulatory system offers a spiritual lesson too. After the lungs oxygenate the blood, the heart pumps the first, best, and freshest blood back to itself. The heart has learned and instructs us in the lesson that "charity begins at home." Serving others is a key part of yoga and loving and caring for ourselves and our own bodies are essential to serve others well. Follow your heart. In all ways give your best energy to your own heart.

## The Respiratory System

Breath occupies a central role in Hatha yoga, both in the practice of asanas and as its own field of practice, pranayama—the control of breath and energy. Breathing capacity is proportional to the ability to control the breath and to the strength and flexibility of the thoracic area.

If chest, ribs, and intercostals are stiff, and if we are unable to fully utilize the diaphragm, breathing capacity is limited. Yoga brings flexibility to, gives fine control over, and increases the capacity of the respiratory system. Yogis have shown that health, vitality, longevity, and mental and emotional states are directly related to the breath. These relationships are discussed in more depth in the section on pranayama in Chapter 5.

## The Digestive System and the Eliminative System

The digestive fire is stoked and toned by exercise. Appetite and the ability to digest foods are greatly increased after exercise. Inverted poses, twists, and forward bends increase the flow of energy to the digestive and eliminative systems, both by directing energy toward these organs and by releasing compression in the spine to increase nerve flow to the digestive organs. Yoga also brings great attention to diet and nutrition. Eating a clean, healthy diet, free from harmful chemicals and toxins, is part of maintaining the digestive and eliminative systems.

Pumping bodily fluids through the body with exercise aids the vital internal organs—kidneys, liver, intestines—in their work. The skin is the largest organ of elimination. Exercise and sweating help the skin eliminate toxins and take the load off other organs. Yoga also uses forward bends, twists, abdominal lifts and churning, and internal cleansing practices to stimulate peristalsis, elimination, and "to keep things moving."

Health is often judged by the externals of muscle tone, strength, and endurance. But the foundation of health lies in the organs of assimilation and elimination. Yoga practice works toward the health of internal organs not only through the benefits of asana practice but also directly through lifestyle, internal cleansing *kriyas,* and by encouraging a clean and healthy diet. It is very important to be attentive to our food intake and to learn the constant, lifelong process of tuning and honing our diets for optimal wellness.

## The Endocrine System

The endocrine glands of the hormonal system affect all aspects of growth, development, and function in the body. Hormones are complex and mysterious chemical messengers that transfer information and instructions between cells. They regulate our mood, tissue function, metabolism, and sexual function, pregnancy, and other reproductive processes. Asana practice, especially inversions, backbends, twists, and breath control, are believed to have strong, beneficial effects on keeping the endocrine system in balance.

After I had been teaching only a few months, one of my first students began having difficulty with her metabolism and energy level after a couple weeks of practice. She told me she was on thyroid medication and I recalled that the Shoulderstand was said to help regulate the thyroid. She was doing a five-minute Shoulderstand each day. I suggested that she have her doctor check her thyroid again. Her doctor found that her thyroid had become more active and was able to reduce her medication. This occurred a couple more times over the months until she was able to go off the medication entirely. This example may be exceptional, but many other cases have shown yoga to help bring mood, energy, and metabolism into a more satisfactory balance.

## The Nervous System

The nervous system is a vast network that conducts vital information throughout the body and consists of the brain, spinal cord, nerves, ganglia, and parts of the receptor and effector organs. Yogis pay special attention to the nerves in the spinal cord, which is seen as part of and an extension of the brain. Nerves traveling through the spinal cord control and affect many organs and muscle systems. These nerves exit the spine through small openings called spinal foramina. As disks and ligaments wear, these openings get smaller and can restrict the flow of energy through the nerves to the corresponding muscles or organs. When we see elderly people walking with canes, often the weakness in their knees and leg muscles is a sign that nerve flow from the spinal cord has been impinged.

Asana practice works to lengthen the spine, maintaining and giving more space to the nerves. Nerve flow can also be improved by breathing and by the practice of directing energy flows along the nerve channels through the use of imagery, intention, sensate awareness, and even by subtle movement in the intended part of the body. In asanas like the Seated Boat, and in standing poses like Half Moon and Balancing Warrior, learning to direct and extend nerve energy out to our extremities, especially into the toes, will keep the nerves active and alive. Yogis can develop a lot of control over their nervous system and can learn to manipulate displaced nerves back into their proper channels. Learning to energize the nerves to keep all parts of the body active and dynamic improves mental capacity, attention, and mental power.

## The Pranic Energy System

In earlier stages of learning Hatha yoga, more attention is placed on physical aspects of the posture such as position, strength, and flexibility. Simply put, in the beginning we are mainly concerned with how to get into a pose and, just as important, how to get out of it. With progress, we begin to develop more awareness of subtler levels.

*Prana* (prah nuh) refers to life force and to subtle flows of energy. Learning to create and direct flows of energy is essential in yoga and in learning inner control, self-healing, and self-development. We discuss the energy body and the breath more extensively in later chapters.

## The Mental-Emotional Systems

Many practitioners consider Hatha yoga to be primarily a mental discipline directed toward the understanding and expansion of consciousness. Developing mental awareness, mental clarity, and insight are at the core of yoga. Although Hatha practice is very physical, it involves a great deal of mental conditioning and development. We learn to expand our attention to all areas of the body while simultaneously directing focus to specific parts. This ability improves powers of mind. Concentration, mental fortitude, and endurance are developed by holding difficult asanas for long periods. Discipline and strength of character come from creating and maintaining a regular practice and all of these qualities are carried over into other areas of life.

The mind and emotions affect one another and are closely related. It has been shown that the nervous and muscular systems store emotional tension and trauma. Massage therapists and body workers often assist their clients in releasing stored emotional tension. Yoga practice is self-directed body work that releases these stored gestalts.

CHAPTER 4

Finding the *Ah Ha!*
in Hatha—Principles,
Hints, and Insights
into Yoga Practice

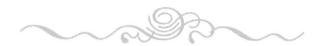

The principles, hints, and insights shared here have been gathered and distilled from many years of study and teaching. I hope that they inspire broadening perspectives and open doors to new levels of possibility in asana practice. These insights and the perspectives they invite can be applied to learning Hatha yoga and they are applicable to many other areas of life as well. They are offered to enrich and add new dimensions and nuances to your yoga experience.

## Presence: Start Where You Are

> Time is the movement from timeless to
> timeless within timelessness.

ATTRIBUTED TO ARISTOTLE

One of the first questions yoga teachers hear from new students is, "How long will it take?" The question not only refers to how much time will be necessary for practice, but also to how long it will take to actually learn and master yoga. Time has been called the poverty of our era. The hurried pace of modern life drives us to feel we have little time for the things we want or need. Time has always been precious but too often we allow our lives to become frenzied and stressful. The new student wants to know how much time he or she must dedicate, how much of the day this yogic endeavor will require, and how long it will take to reach the goal. I have often answered these questions by saying, "It will take the rest of your life." This is actually good news. Yoga is not a goal at all—it is a lifelong process of living and learning that nurtures our being and that enriches the quality of our days. Realizing the significance of this insight removes unproductive pressures we may otherwise bring to our approach. We have our entire lifetimes.

We will always have much to learn and more to develop in the ways of skill and techniques, but the essence of yoga is deeper—it is always immediate and available as it grows from refining our attunement to the flow of life, and life force. Our bodies constantly change and adjust to our internal and external states, not only day to day but through many stages of a lifetime. That is why a more meaningful practice promises no end but provides a constant journey of learning and discovering. Advancing our practice implies refining our ability to see and listen to our body on deeper and subtler levels. Cultivating this internal perception is more important than merely attaining more exotic postures. We can develop great strength or flexibility but miss the heart of the practice. I have seen some teachers, and even some students, quickly master very difficult and impressive postures. Many of their fellow students regard them with awe as highly advanced yogis. On closer observation it might become apparent that a seemingly advanced yogi may be practicing arrogantly, aggressively, or competitively, with little awareness of the subtle, internal levels of his or her experience in asanas. Someone may be able to twist into a pretzel while balancing on one finger and still be a novice who misses the heart and essence of yoga.

Making the time for a yoga practice means to honor and love ourselves enough to dedicate time each day to our own well-being. Serving ourselves is part of serving others. Only when we take care of ourselves can we have more abundant energy to give to others and to our endeavors. When a student tells me, "I can't find the time to take out of my daily life for practice or exercise," I reply, "Neither can I." They usually look a bit shocked until I explain that I have quite a bit of responsibility with a lot of office work to do, projects and staff to supervise, as well as an occasional crisis to manage. Often it seems there are not enough hours in the day. I don't have time to "take out" for my yoga practice either, and yet I keep up a regular practice. I certainly know that I have much more energy, much more quality time and freedom, and much better health than would have been possible without having allowed myself time for asana. In truth, yoga doesn't "take time"—it gives time.

Can we approach yoga in a way that is free of time constraints and free from unproductive pressures we impose on ourselves? Consider the old saying, "Start where you are and stay there." Pondering the wisdom of this apparent paradox reveals the importance of keeping our attention on the moment and not only on our goals. It reveals the need to be present. Starting where you are implies tuning into your body and accepting and moving from your present state. Staying where you are implies keeping the attention in your asanas on your actual abilities in each moment of your practice. When we first start something we are infused with excitement, energy, and humility; we want to learn, we ask many questions. How do we maintain this beginner's mind? This is the lesson we need to learn from the joy and exuberance of children. When we are young, we are filled with excitement for learning. As our knowledge and experience grow, our attitude begins to crystallize and harden into the state of mind called "I know." All too often the more we know, the less we understand. Knowledge can harden us if we don't keep our quest for insight alive. Keep a beginner's mind—a fresh, questioning approach unburdened by baggage from the past.

## The Long View

Being present is balanced and tempered by keeping a long view, a lifetime perspective. Every body ages. A person twenty years of age is less apt to pay attention to this inevitability than a sixty-year-old, but the earlier we become aware of aging the more we will learn from the process. I was on a swimming team in high school and clearly recall having the thought, at about age fifteen, that if I swam a mile regularly I would be able to swim well and be fit when I was eighty or ninety, so I decided to try. I was fortunate to have this kind of intention early and it greatly increased with the study of Hatha yoga. In the early days of our Los Angeles yoga center, which was on the second floor across from a meeting hall, I would look out the window and watch people arriving and leaving for events. There would be supple, energetic kids running up and down the stairs and playing. Then I'd notice many middle-aged and older folks coming in with stooped shoulders, bent frames, stiff bodies, and worse. I realized that the bodies of the older people were essentially the same as those of the younger people, just a few years later. Without endeavoring, without regular work to maintain strength and flexibility, people can lose their mobility.

How would you act if you received a wonderful new car when you were sixteen years of age but were told that this was to be your only vehicle for your entire lifetime? How would you care for it? Although our bodies change and are self-healing, we do in fact have only one body for our lifetime. Acknowledging this fact and treating the body accordingly is an important part of taking the long view. We are all subject to setbacks from circumstance, accident, injury, or illness. Yogis learn and gather tools to rebalance themselves and to become self-healers. Where will we be ten or twenty years from now if we do not have a personal yoga practice? Many students are concerned or worried that they do not make progress quickly enough. It is actually fairly easy to stay where you are now, maintaining current levels of strength, flexibility, and endurance for many years. Most people would be pretty happy if they could be in the physical condition they are in today twenty years from now. In the long view, even staying in the same place is a great attainment. Young people often push aggressively in their yoga practices and cause long-term, long-lasting injuries. Joints and ligaments can be injured or worn out. Are we practicing in a way that builds and maintains our body's parts or that wears them out? Are we even asking that question? Holding such questions during practice is important. Even if someone fifty, sixty, or seventy years of age just beginning yoga could maintain his or her current level of physical ability for the next quarter century, it would be of great value and benefit. Practice with the long view by holding an entire lifetime in perspective. We need to practice so that, looking back years from now, we'll be content with ourselves.

## The Asanas Are Tools, Not Goals

"Have no goal!" is another common expression we hear attributed to Eastern philosophies. We're told that goals lead to pressure and conflict—between the present actuality and the desired possibility. The message encourages us to live only in the moment, but is this even possible? Deeper questions often end in paradox or, perhaps better said, polarity. Does time exist or is there only eternity? Is light matter or energy? These questions have no single answer. The answer depends on how you look at the question. Should I have goals in my practice or no goals? The answer is yes, to both. We can have goals of strength, endurance, and flexibility. We may want to attain a certain asana or master certain techniques. But underlying the goals a softer core of *non-goal awareness* is needed. We begin to see that our abilities, like all things, wax and wane. The process and constant attunement with the actuality of the moment is more important than any attainment. When goal orientation no longer drives us, we can move from an inner place of being rather than from the harder outer place of doing. It is important to balance *attaining* with *attuning*. We may want to attain a stronger, better asana, but it should not be at the expense of attuning to our body's capabilities in the moment. It is possible to have goals *and* have no goal at the same time.

In addition to balancing our overall goal orientation with an inward approach, we need to consider how we tend to make each asana a goal in and of itself. We see the Lotus pose, a beautiful backbend, or the Headstand, and it becomes our goal to achieve it. This desire can create an aggressive or competitive practice and lead to injury. It is a common mindset to try to power through our weaknesses. I recall an overanxious student who, regardless of all warnings and advice, zealously pushed his legs toward the Lotus posture. He would sit with his foot on his thigh, alternately bouncing each of his knees down to loosen his hips. Then he would force his legs into the posture, sitting with a winced smile on his face for the two seconds he could maintain it. Eventually he injured his knees and it was years before he healed and could do the pose again. Sometimes going slower is going faster.

Another lesson we can learn when we begin to see yoga practices and asanas as tools is that we need to learn the proper and skillful use of these tools. It is important to understand that asana practice isn't automatically beneficial. Yoga practices can heal, but they can also injure. Although they are predominantly benign and in most cases beneficial, it is more intelligent to be aware of potential harm and endeavor to increase our skills in the personal application of yoga.

Asanas are tools, used to work on our bodies, to heal or to build strength, flexibility, and endurance, much more than asanas are goals. They are also great metaphors to see our nature, our character, and the ways we move through life. *The asanas are tools and their purpose is to serve our body, mind, and spirit.* They are not just goals to be attained. A story of a famous tailor in India named Hamsa-ji illustrates this point. One day Hamsa-ji was in a hurry to leave his shop when a customer, walking tall, came in to buy a suit. He said he must have the suit right away so he could wear it for a special occasion that very evening. Hamsa-ji pulled out a suit and gave it to the man to try on. The man quickly slipped into the suit and stood before the tailor in front of a mirror. The right leg and left arm were a bit too long and the jacket seemed large, so the man asked that they be fixed, but it was late and Hamsa-ji had no time. "The problem is all in your posture!" asserted the tailor. He instructed his customer, "Please lift your chest, now drop your right shoulder a little. Good. Now, please, raise your right hip when you walk. Look in the mirror now, my dear sir. Does this suit fit or does it not?" The man smiled at his contorted figure in the mirror. The suit was a perfect fit, so he happily paid Hamsa-ji and hobbled out of the shop in his new outfit and new posture. A couple of the neighboring shopkeepers were chatting in the street as he left. One commented, "Brother, look at that poor cripple. Only Hamsa-ji, the great tailor, could fit a man like that!" We shouldn't try to cram ourselves into asanas like Hamsa-ji did to that man; rather, we can learn how to use and adjust the asanas to our needs.

Postures and practice should be adjusted to the needs and levels of each practitioner, not the other way around. Yet more often than not, students approach limitations in reverse and force themselves into postures. It is said that there are 840,000 asanas. In one way this mythic figure is a metaphor for a flexible approach to finding the appropriate poses for particular purposes, as it suggests there is a variation or adjustment of every pose for any body. Goals have their place. They give us energy and move us forward. They give purpose and direction and motivate us to achieve. However, focusing excessively on goals can cause aggressive practice that takes us out of the moment and out of attunement to the journey. Softening our goal orientation can help overcome aggressiveness and effort in yoga practice so we are more able to enjoy the journey. Goals are the finish line of a race, while yoga is an ongoing process throughout life. We need goals, and we need to keep them in their place.

## Feedback: Learning to Listen

External learning and observation must be balanced with awakening an internal awareness. Yoga brings our attention to both the inner and outer aspects of our being. An important part of inner attention is learning to listen to the intelligence that lives in the body. Though it may not speak in words, the body communicates loudly and clearly when we listen. It will teach correct movements and point out mistakes, singing when we work hard and asking for rest too. The body's myriad feedback loops resonate together at higher levels of complexity. In the same way we watch how nature's systems interrelate and affect each other, we can learn to monitor the relational effects of our body's internal systems. Our breathing affects the mind, our thoughts affect the immune system, what we eat affects our mood, physical activity affects emotions, and so on and on. Watching these interactions and learning to work with them is an important part of the inner process of yogic development.

Looking back on an experience I had as a teen helped me to understand this. I had just turned sixteen and made friends with an older, more experienced kid who had just moved to town from Detroit. We went together to the house of a young girl my friend was trying to woo. She pulled out a cigarette and he whipped out his metal lighter and, with a practiced movement, opened it, quickly gave her a light, and snapped it shut with a loud metallic click. Then he got out his pack of Marlboros, popped one in his mouth, and offered me one. "You smoke, don't you?" he asked. "Of course," I replied, having never had a puff in my life. He lit our cigarettes with the same snapping movements, and I was really impressed. I took a deep drag of smoke. To this day I remember the nausea, the room spinning around, and the intense urge to choke and cough. I would love to see the expression on my face as I sat there using every ounce of will power to fight off the sensations and look cool as I took repeated drags.

What I later learned was that my body was telling me in every way it could that this was a toxic substance. It screamed, it shouted, it sent coughs and mucus, but I fought back, saying essentially, "Shut up!" So in a short time it gave up and stopped using energy to shout on deaf ears. Instead, it adjusted by creating the inner systems necessary to process the toxic, new chemicals. This is how the addiction process works. I went on to eventually smoke a pack of cigarettes a day until one day, a couple of years into college, I took a fresh look at my habit. With the same will power I used to fake it before, I threw my cigarettes in the trash, never to smoke again. Our bodies can teach us and speak to us (as silly as that may sound). When we do not listen, the body stops wasting energy and just adjusts to our bad habits. When we begin to live more sensitively and to watch and tune in, the body will tentatively begin giving us feedback again and the process reverses. Our own bodies can become our most important teachers. When watching and listening to feedback, it is important to pay attention to the immediate effects as well as intermediate and long-term effects of the practices. We keep an eye on how our practice affects us in the moment, what the effects are the next day, and several days later. We may not be able to see all the effects exactly or specifically, but staying as attentive as possible will go a long way.

I also learned a lot about listening from an Indian yogi in Europe. The yogi was not an advanced Hatha practitioner by ordinary measures—the ability to perform feats of strength or flexibility—but he was truly a master of more important levels of yogic practice. He pointed out that we must balance the inner voice with our intellectual knowledge. One morning he came into the room where we were all going to practice together, did a few stretches, sat for a few minutes, and then got up and left. At lunch I asked him what happened. He said that he felt tired and uninspired so he took a look at it. He "asked his body," which he said replied that it had a hard and very physical day yesterday with lots of interviews and it needed rest now more than work.

He also pointed out that this message could be a sign of laziness so one must look at all levels of feedback and think them through. We should make use of all the capacities available to us, including our minds, intellectual knowledge, and the internal feedback from the body's intelligence. It is millions of years old, which gives it seniority even to tradition.

The yogi's behavior contrasts sharply with another experience I had. When traveling I visited a teacher well known for being a strict disciplinarian and for an uncompromising approach. After a morning class he took written questions in a formal way, without any dialogue or interaction. I asked him what he thought of listening to the body's intelligence. What should we do if one morning we feel our body is telling us to take it easy or take rest? His brow furrowed and he got fiery and intense. He said that he couldn't believe a "senior" yoga teacher would ask a question like this. He said that if he started his practice and his body told him to rest, he would do a double practice that day. He didn't ask his body what to do, he *told* his body what to do. Perhaps there are times when an approach like his can be valuable—and it is safer in youth—but in a lifelong practice a more cooperative relationship yields better fruit. There is also another big difference in the two teachers. One is open-minded, willing to listen and dialogue showing humor, happiness, and self-actualization; the other is somewhat self-righteous, authoritarian, and irritable. I do not know which came first, the attitude or the approach, but certainly a rigid practice did not help to soften the second yogi. So I recommend that we learn to work with the balance of control and surrender, internal feedback and external information, and the myriad other polarities in life.

## Strength and Flexibility

An important aspect of working with physical polarities is to understand the interplay of strength and flexibility. Our bodies require healthy integration of both in the right balance to function properly. When yoga first arrived in the West, it generated an enormous fascination with flexibility, probably due to the exotic pretzel contortions the early yogis demonstrated. Even now, many people associate yoga with flexibility postures. When I mention that I do yoga, a common response is, "Yes, I do some stretching too." Or conversely, "I can't do yoga, I'm too stiff." A yoga practice involves far more than merely being limber. When I first learned Hatha yoga, a great emphasis was put on flexibility. My teacher, a respected yogi from India, rarely emphasized building strength. Instead he focused primarily on attaining the difficult pretzel poses, which were said to have mysterious and mystical benefits. I was an athlete and already fairly strong, but I was very stiff, so the strange positions from India were attractive. We were taught about subtle energies and strange forces, and I didn't think that the principles I had learned in sports applied here. Warming up was considered "stretching out" before getting into deeper poses. We rested and cooled down after each position. The major emphasis was "to attain the asana and get the benefits." After a few years of practicing this way, I started to have back pains, neck pains, and eventually serious injuries. It took some time to analyze what was wrong and begin to correct it.

As we have seen, the syllable *Ha* in *Hatha* means sun, which implies masculine energy and symbolizes heating, expansion, and strength; *Tha* means moon, which refers to feminine energy and symbolizes cooling, contraction, and flexibility. It is vitally important to bring these principles into balance. Too much flexibility and cooling can be as problematic as too much strength. Flexibility without strength leads to fragility. Strength without flexibility leads to rigidity. As you practice, become attuned to the relationship of these principles and aware of which principle needs emphasis. Women tend to need to work a little harder on strength, men on flexibility, but the balance of the two changes in each person each day. If I have been doing a lot of hiking and strenuous physical activities, then I usually have a softer practice with more flexibility work to restore equilibrium. When I have been sedentary, my practice is more vigorous and dynamic. Don't hold your poses too rigidly, with too much *Ha,* or too passively with too much *Tha.* Watching the interaction of strength and flexibility is one of the things that holds my interest and keeps my practice fresh.

## Heating and Cooling

Watching the principles of sun and moon also teaches us to balance heating and cooling. My first teacher somehow omitted this important concept. He either did not know about it or, perhaps, being from the hot climate of India where properly warming the muscles is less critical, he overlooked it. On many days rather than warming up, we would start our practice by simply stretching cold muscles until they loosened, and then we would move on to stronger work. We were told to rest after every posture, which cooled us down again. When I began to see the problems caused by practicing cold and moving hard muscles too quickly, I learned to warm up properly and to stay warm, and soon discovered that it took less time to loosen warm muscles.

Warm muscles stretch farther and easier with increased circulation, greater strength, and less risk of injury. Don't confuse stretching with warming up. A warm-up is one of the basic stages of any standard physical workout, yet many yoga students do not include it. Exactly what it sounds like, a warm-up is an activity to get the body warm and soft, with increased circulation. Move carefully into postures while you are cold. Avoid going to your normal maximum until the body complies easily. Slowly increase your movements as the muscles become warm and pliable. I generally do not recommend resting between poses either, except in instances where a short rest is needed after an intense pose or in specific cases such as hypertension, illness, or old age. Many poses may be used to warm up, but Sun Salutations or a series of standing positions are often the best. Ease into them, staying well short of your maximum edges or going only to your minimum edge—where you first feel stiffness or resistance. With each successive repetition, with each breath, you will slowly and effortlessly move deeper and more fully into the posture. Finally, make sure you stay warm during the practice until you begin the cool-down phase. You will have more energy, increased benefits, and greater enjoyment.

Physically generated heat can also purify and detoxify our bodies. The skin is the largest organ of elimination. When we get hot during practice, the increased circulation filters more blood through our organs and the increased heat also allows detoxifying through sweating. These conditions allow a sort of burning, washing, and breathing out of toxins. This detoxification occurs whether or not we physically sweat, but there is a unique type of high and feeling of release of tension after a workout in which we break a sweat. Some students hold onto the erroneous concept that we should not work hard or sweat in yoga. They might confuse working the body with straining it. "Never strain," they say. This is true, but strain means to overexert or go beyond your limits. Pain, shaking, or too much "efforting" evidences straining. Don't confuse the principle of not straining with not working. We can work very hard and still not strain.

Some believe that sweating or working hard may be appropriate for gymnastics or calisthenics but not for yoga. This is a foolish notion. Conversely, some teachers assert that you must work hard, sweat, and generate lots of internal heat in every session or you are not practicing properly. "No pain, no gain," they may say. This approach, while energizing and invigorating, can also lead to imbalances. Practitioners who work with too much heat can develop a strained look about them. They sometimes have bags or circles under their eyes or look gaunt from the stress of too much heat. Nature does not behave in this single-minded way. Everything in nature moves in cycles, always balancing itself—inner to outer to inner, heating to cooling and then to heating, winter into spring, and on into summer into fall. The extremes of sweating all the time or of never working hard enough to sweat both miss the subtlety of learning to work with the balance of hot and cold in the organism. Either principle, hot or cold, can be overemphasized and brought out of balance. Each of the various ways to practice yoga has its appropriate place and time.

Once on a trip deep into the Himalayas, I finally caught up with a renowned magical yogi I had heard about for years. He had enormous charisma and seemed to have the power to know people from the inside. He was staying at a temple, and being a fire yogi, he sat by the sacred fire surrounded by many exotic *sadhus,* or renunciate wanderers. They would sing and chant beautiful ancient texts together for hours a day, making wonderful music and creating an extraordinary sight. I sat for a day and a half just observing the scene, and he never once looked at or seemed to notice me in the crowd. Finally, I decided I was ready to go up and meet him. At that exact moment he swung around in his chair, looked right at me, smiled mischievously, and waved me toward him. I went up, said "Namaste," and we exchanged some greetings. He asked me what I did in America. I hesitated, anticipating his response in the midst of this extraordinary gathering of fakirs and yogis. But I stuck my neck out and said I was a yoga teacher. He gave me another bizarre look and said, "Okay, go give a yoga class to those men over there!" He pointed to a circle of the glorious and frightening men. They were mountain yogis, many of whom lived in Himalayan caves. Some had long matted locks piled on their heads, some were naked, some smeared in ashes from the sacred fire. They were muscular and severe looking, but friendly. They were yogis who had mastered the inner heat principle and could live in the freezing cold without clothing, going days without food. His message was obvious. There is much more to yoga than only the surface practices.

## The Rhythms and Seasons of Practice

We do not have to sit naked in the Himalayas to master yoga, but the Hatha yoga student would do well to learn about the play of opposites represented by the sun and moon. Start with something as simple as learning about heating and cooling in your body. Our practice needs to work with balancing these energies. A practice of yoga might cycle like the seasons. All things move in cycles of change. Spring brings blossom and growth. Summer brings more light and nourishment. The inner flows and expresses itself outwardly. In the fall, energy is gathered and stored, and in winter, reserves are used and inner processes dominate. The changing cycle of seasons in nature can inspire and guide our practice. Our bodies move through seasons of change from childhood to old age. The seasons of our practice change with the natural seasons, in subcycles of their own and in the cycles of life from youth to old age.

Our process of yoga can grow and adjust with the cycles and subcycles of living. This suggests tuning into the rhythms in the body. Many changes occur within us each day as well as from week to week. We do not live in just one season either, so we must think and feel beyond just the calendar. In the winter, we heat our homes; in the summer, we use shade and cooling. Similarly, our practice always involves a mixture and interplay of many opposites. Sometimes we need more Ha, or sun, type sessions that are stronger, more vigorous workouts. At other times we need the moon, or softer, more relaxing sessions. No fixed formula dictates which to do when; only the subjective process of learning to listen and balance can guide us to self-healing. When we understand and do not resist, our bodies want to move toward balance. Remaining in extremes actually creates the difficulties. Nature will always throw us back from an extreme to the middle or to the other, opposite pole. The body's intelligence often finds its own way to stop excess. Paying attention to sun and moon, hot and cold, and their ever-changing cycles will help in learning the balance of yoga.

## Tension Is Your Friend

Muscular tension is necessary. The body constantly adjusts and changes its levels of muscle tension to support the skeletal structure, to protect the joints, and to absorb shock. The musculature of the body acts on the skeletal system like a series of interrelated springs and tensions that are constantly resetting each other at levels appropriate to the particular activities we engage in. These "springs" are composed of multiple processes of varying tensions, strengths, flexibilities, and hard and soft structures. Tensions interact and combine in many variations to reach higher levels of order and performance.

Stiffness is not a hostile adversary; rather, it is the operation of intelligence in the body. It is probably more appropriate to think in terms of keeping tension in the right balance than of eliminating it. A construction worker needs a different balance from that of a dancer. Hard work carrying lumber and bricks strengthens and hardens the musculature in different relationships than a dancer might desire. When we hike or do heavy work, the body naturally tightens. When we sit for a long time, the body adjusts its tensions accordingly. When we stand up and walk after sitting for a long time, we feel stiff. What we're feeling is residual stiffness from the previous activity dissipating as the body resets its tensions for the new activity. If we do not keep the muscles pliable and able to reset, we may create imbalances that result in stiffness, pain, immobility, or lack of skeletal alignment.

Both our activities and our inactivities affect the tension balance in our bodies. One purpose of yoga practice is to keep limits of strength, flexibility, tightness, and softness malleable and transformable. Broadening the limits of flexibility and the body's capacity to adjust is one of the purposes—and effects—of the asanas. Yoga practice leads to spring tensions that are more easily set and changed and can reach the right balance for the lifestyle we lead. Simply put, with a regular yoga practice, the body can more easily restore equilibrium after stiffening from hard work, strenuous physical activity, or even from periods of inactivity.

## Inner- and Outer-Directed Practices

Asana practices can be divided into two broad categories. The first includes "outer-directed" practices that follow a specific form, sequence, or structure. The Flow Series we teach is an example of this type. Outer-directed practices have many advantages. These series are balanced sessions that give the benefits of proper sequencing, many types of poses, and complete practices. Fixed sequences allow us to flow through our practice with concentration and awareness, without having to figure out what to do next. We can also more easily gauge our progress— many feel improvement is made more rapidly by regularly following well-designed, fixed sequences. The second category, "inner-directed," refers to practices that are more intuitive. They are designed more specifically for an individual or are created by the practitioner by attuning to the needs of the moment. The practice may vary each day, and one endeavors to listen, respond, and adjust to the specific feedback from within.

Some adherents to fixed sequences say their teachings have remained unchanged since great souls or "masters" revealed them in ancient times. Unquestioning belief in the perfection of a system can be a key ingredient in a recipe for abuse and authoritarianism. Usually these "perfect" systems can be easily disproved, if the adherents will even listen to other points of view. Fixed practices may not be open to growth, evolution, or feedback. Those who believe solely in the intuitive approach argue that fixed sequences are rigid and inappropriate because they force the person into the system rather than adjusting the system to each individual. But those who practice solely in an intuitive manner miss the unique benefits of following a well-designed fixed sequence.

Inner-directed practice and outer-directed practice are two sides of an equation that are related to and balance each other. Both methods can also overlap and contain each other. For example, if you are practicing a fixed sequence, you can still do so in an intuitive way within the sequence. You are listening to your body and adjusting the poses, their intensity, length of time, and other factors uniquely in the moment. Similarly, if you are practicing and creating an intuitive, inner-directed sequence, you still use the forms, structures, and rules of asana practice.

Both types of practice are unique and useful—I use both of them. There have been periods of months and even a few years where I practiced essentially the same sequence of poses as an experiment or because I was deriving particular benefits. I learned never to tire of the regimen because, even though the sequence was the same, my experiences of it in my body were different each time. The subtleties and nuances changed during each session. At one point I even realized, only half humorously, that I had "never practiced in a body this old before" and that this in fact was true every day. My attention focused on how I was feeling and the effects of the poses. I suggest you take advantage of both options. There are days when following a fixed series may be just what the doctor ordered, and other days where going with the flow is the order of the day. Why limit yourself to one or the other when both have unique benefits and appropriateness?

## Mental Limitations

Yoga requires mental practice as much as it involves physical discipline. A student of yoga always seeks to learn physically, mentally, and spiritually. Our minds can limit our practice as much as our bodies do.

The body may have ability and energy but the mind can easily become bored, lazy, or distracted. That is why involving and using one's mind and attention are at the core of yoga practice. The concepts we hold about ourselves can be real stumbling blocks. We form these concepts and beliefs and continually reinforce them through word and thought. Many students repeat negative statements such as, "I get tired easily," "I have no discipline," or "I have terrible balance." These assertions may have some truth, but constantly repeating them like mantras only strengthens them. The power of mind cuts both ways. I have been able to assist students in moving through blocks or inabilities simply by getting them to say, "I have the energy to do it," or "I am learning to do this pose."

Even positive self-images create problems. We may approach our practice with a concept of what we can or should be able to do, or of what we have done in the past. By focusing on the concept or memory instead of on our actual ability in the moment, we may push too far. I have seen this undesirable tendency not only with people trying to do today what they know they could do yesterday, but in longer cycles too. Many times someone wants to get into shape after years of neglect. Though it has been a long time since they had a physical practice, it might seem like only yesterday, so they push too hard at first. This tendency can be more serious for older people and seniors. It is difficult to accept our decline, and too often a seventy-year-old tries to his or her detriment to keep up with a twenty-five-year-old in the same class. *Start where you are and stay there.* Watch your mental projections, images, and concepts and use them wisely. Positive self-images, when tempered with reality, can bring inspiration and energy.

## Fear As a Limitation

Fear can prevent students from moving forward or from doing certain postures. Inverted poses such as Headstand or Handstand and more difficult backbends and other poses that challenge strength and balance commonly cause some people to tense up or shy away.

Most fear in yoga practice is created by anticipation and by projecting thought forward. In the moment of true danger there is actually no fear, only reaction or action. If you are crossing the street and suddenly a car comes at you seemingly out of nowhere, you immediately jump out of the way. The fear comes afterwards when you think about what could have happened and your heart races. Or the fear comes the next time you go to cross that street and you think about or anticipate what might happen.

This same kind of fear reaction can occur when learning a difficult position. The deep instincts we have of fight or flight cause us to send many signals coursing through our nervous systems that tense and stimulate the muscles. Fear also comes from our unfamiliarity with how to execute a new and challenging pose. Our uncertainty results in tensing or energizing many muscle sets at once instead of only the necessary ones. This excessive effort can sap energy and even cause strain or injury. Many times when teaching more challenging postures, I see the student's body become hard, rigid, and heavier than normal. When I explain this process, students learn to soften and relax as they explore new positions.

## Competition and Comparison

Yoga teachers often say that we should practice without competition and comparison to others. On closer examination, we see it is really neither possible nor desirable to do this. We constantly compare ourselves to more and less advanced students, to our teachers, to the "ideal" pose, and to what we can or want to be able to do. These comparisons contribute greatly to the learning process. Even if we try to practice only for our own well-being or excellence, that intention itself involves subtle forms of comparison and competition. A better connotation of the advice not to compete nor compare suggests we take pressure off of ourselves by releasing our thoughts of inferiority or superiority in our practice. Your practice is for you—for your growth, development, and well-being.

Yoga is a field where everyone can win, because winning is not about who does the best asana but about learning to do the best asana for your body in each moment. The usual competition with others for a prize or recognition is not involved and so comparison has no relevance except for the purpose of learning. Watching a more advanced student can be a source of inspiration and instruction. Practice to learn and grow, not to win or defeat. Yoga is one of the few arenas in which everyone wins.

## Yoga Is for Every Body

Many people have fixed ideas about what physical body type is suitable for yoga practice. Remember, asanas are tools we learn to use to maintain our well-being, and that among the legendary 840,000 postures there is certainly something for everyone. In my years of teaching I've seen people with virtually every type of body learn and benefit from yoga. I've had the opportunity to teach the tall, short, fat, thin, weak, and disabled. I've seen quadriplegics benefit from doing only the breathing techniques. I met a teacher who began bedridden with paralysis, started only with breathing, progressed to walking, and eventually mastered many postures. There is no perfect yoga body—yoga is perfect for every body. Nature in her wisdom creates myriad forms and none have overall superiority. The Adonis body may be best suited for one task and the weakling another. It takes all kinds.

When I opened my first center, the Center for Yoga in Los Angeles, the very first student through the door was a man named Charles Hobby. I didn't know then that Charlie was to become an important teacher for me. He was a court reporter, the best in town, with his choice of all the top trials. I was twenty-one and he was forty years old, short and stocky with a great deal of stiffness aggravated by the necessity to sit and type for at least ten hours a day. "I am very stiff and I sit all day. Will I be able to get flexible and do all those poses if I practice diligently?" he asked. "Of course," I replied with conviction, for I had heard many testimonials and anecdotes from my teachers. I had only been teaching a few months when he arrived. I must admit I had plenty of doubts, but I didn't want to discourage him. "I'll do it," he said, "as long as I don't have to get into spiritual mumbo jumbo."

Charlie practiced more regularly than any student I had known. He took pride in attending class every day, six days a week. When he started he couldn't touch his toes and he could hardly twist. Backbends were but a distant hope. His progress was barely noticeable for a long while, but he started getting benefits right away. His tension, aches, and pains diminished by the day, so he kept on. He would often ask if he really would ever attain the flexibility to get into the most basic postures. After several months he could touch his toes. After a year and a half he could fold in half in his forward bends. He was elated and radiant. Now he was asking if he could ever do the Lotus and backbends. Again I answered in the affirmative, with my lingering inner doubts. In a few more years Charlie was doing the Wheel and Camel backbends. I'll never forget the day he walked in front of the class, smiled, and slowly pulled his legs into the Lotus posture. I looked at him that day and realized it was as if he had reincarnated into a different body from the one he came in the door with years earlier. He was still short and stout, but now he was muscular, leaner, and he had a glow around him. He was full of health and vitality and his aches and pains were now the distant memory. To my astonishment, Charlie then announced that he wanted to learn about meditation and the spiritual aspects of yoga. Getting the stiffness out of his body changed his outlook. Now he could also bend his mind. Charlie taught me the power of patience and per-severance and showed me that all things are possible.

# There Is No Such Thing as Perfection

We have a natural tendency to create and project images and goals of perfection. Some branches of Eastern philosophy even describe attaining perfection as the goal of life. Seeking perfection can be counterproductive in one's yoga practice. It can bring struggle and conflict. I had the good fortune to study science and physics in college, and I learned a principle then that proved useful when applied to life. In a sense, there is actually no such thing as perfection. We can create mathematical equations for a straight line, a perfect circle, or a perfect sphere. But in reality these perfect forms do not exist. There are no straight lines, no perfect circles nor perfect spheres in nature. In fact, space is curved and time is warped. Although we perceive linearity in nature, upon closer inspection or by breaking physical measures down to the lower levels, we find deviations from linearity. Everything seems to contain at least small imperfections. Even evolution, it is interesting to note, progresses through error, mutation, and selection.

A look at art also underlines this insight. The most striking art is full of imperfection. The most boring art is a dull reproduction. If you tuned a piano to perfect frequencies, an exact octave, for example, it would sound dissonant and some say it might damage the instrument. That is why piano tuners have to seek the slight imperfections in the frequencies so chords and octaves sound right to the imperfect human ear.

We waste too much energy projecting images of perfection and trying to live up to unattainable goals. We beat ourselves up too easily with expectations we create of how we *should be* in our postures and in our lives. It is a natural tendency to envision an idealized pose and then work—or worse, struggle—to attain it. Unfortunately, our efforts at perfection can be counterproductive and can take us away from being in tune with the needs and actualities of the moment. It may be more fruitful simply to tune in to our own needs and levels of ability, not push ourselves unreasonably, and to work within our limits. But here paradox raises its head again because it is also important to work on improvement and to use the examples of more advanced students and more refined postures to motivate and guide us. Sometimes pushing oneself onward and exerting a bit more can lead to breakthroughs and leaps in ability. The bottom line again is sensitivity, balance, and learning to listen to know what will be most productive and healthful. Understanding what natural laws show about perfection can guide us as we learn through our own errors and it may help us to lighten up on ourselves a bit. This understanding may apply usefully to other areas of life too. Looking back, we see that some of our greatest lessons came from our errors. If everything is perfection, then imperfection is part of the process, part of the perfection of all things.

## Discipline

I often hear students say, "I don't have the discipline to keep up a regular practice. I really would like to but somehow I'm just not disciplined enough." Does this sound familiar? People often comment about how disciplined I seem to be. I actually don't feel disciplined at all, at least in the usual sense of the word. We often hold discipline to mean the effort to do certain things we think we need to do, or should be doing, but in fact we don't have the energy or will to do. Where do we get the energy, then? When we are really interested in something or really enjoying something, we do not need what we call discipline to do it. In fact, the root meaning of the word comes from *discere,* which means *to learn.* I've learned to enjoy my practice and to keep it fresh and interesting. I do this by following my interests, approaching each session freshly, and by not beating myself up when I don't feel like working. Staying in touch with the benefits, energy, and well-being that my practice gives me is what keeps my energy flowing.

Developing regularity in our practice is very important, but regularity differs dramatically from routine and regimentation. It is more important to be free, open, and responsive to the needs of each moment than to have a regimented daily practice. At the same time, we need to avoid irregularity and sporadic practice. Routine or regimentation can imply a rote, mechanical process that soon becomes boring and tiring. Staying in tune with the process and benefits you experience keeps energy to practice flowing. We can become hooked, in a positive sense, on feeling good, strong, and flexible. If, due to circumstances, we miss too many days, we will begin to notice undesirable differences in our bodies and this awareness will give us the energy to get going again.

Taking time off occasionally, by choice or necessity, allows the body to rest and heal. I take at least one day a week off and find this aspect of my practice very beneficial. But it isn't necessary to schedule my day off—circumstances provide it. Many times after intentionally or inadvertently missing a few days, I come back stronger and *more* flexible. In a lifelong practice, even the down times become part of the process and learning experience. Don't beat yourself up for missing some days, but also don't develop the habit of being "regularly irregular." I have witnessed people so fanatical about their routines that they miss out on many of the joys of living. I recall traveling with a yoga teacher who missed a beautiful tour of a foreign city and a sunset cruise on a river because he wouldn't skip his morning practice. My practice that morning was the adventure and my yoga lost nothing.

It is also important, especially for newer students, to develop and maintain a momentum or constancy of practice. Building a strong foundation through periods of consistent dedication carries us through the lean times when we cannot practice and helps establish a lifelong practice. We can learn to see our practice as an opportunity instead of a chore. We can see our practice as a journey in which we are always learning and make the shift from saying, "I have to do my yoga" to "I get to do my yoga."

## Concentration and Attention

Concentration means focusing awareness toward one point. A story about the great warrior-archer, Arjuna, tells how he and some fellow students were being taught how to shoot the bow to hit an apple on a post. The teacher asked the first student what he saw as he drew his bow. He described the mountain scene, the post, and the apple. The second student described the post and how the apple was sitting on it. Arjuna's turn came and, as he drew his bow back and took aim, his teacher asked what he saw. "I only see the apple," he replied as he let go of the arrow and sliced the target in half. That is concentration. Attention is different: it is broader, more inclusive, contextual, and not limited to one activity. Attention implies awareness of many things at once. A mother can be speaking on the phone and cooking a meal, but she is still aware of her baby's every sound.

In the early stages of Hatha practice we have difficulty staying aware of everything required in a posture. There is breathing, specific alignments, movement of musculature, and energy. Concentration by its very nature has to move from point to point. Students often find that as they concentrate on one point, they lose another. The legs are energized and aligned and the arms go limp, for example. After some practice and progress, concentration begins expanding into a more all-encompassing attention. Be careful, though: If attention is forced, it becomes concentration. During your asana practice, you should develop a quality of attention that is naturally aware of every part of your body, the flow of energy, your breathing, alignment, and even the room you are in. Students will learn to keep all parts of their body active, alive, and energized in the pose. Once this ability is developed, it is even possible to simultaneously concentrate on one area of the body without diminishing *attention*. This exercise in awareness and focus helps increase the powers of mind.

## Using the Breath

The breath, like attention and awareness, is central to your practice. The quality and manner of breathing have a great effect on the character of the practice. While the breath may be used many ways, the main point is to become aware of your breathing while you practice—watching the quality of breathing and endeavoring to keep it smooth, even, and rhythmic. This process will bring these same qualities to the postures and movements. Let breath flow freely while equalizing and creating a balance between inhalations and exhalations. Most of the time it is best to breathe through the nostrils instead of the mouth. The nasal passages filter and warm the air, absorb more pranic energy, and help balance the sun and moon energies of the body.

Inhalation increases energy while tightening and strengthening, while exhalation releases energy, softening and lengthening. We can use this biomechanical understanding of the breath in the poses. For example, in a forward bend you can use the strengthening of inhalation to help lift the chest and elongate the spinal cord, and then use the softening of exhalation to stretch farther forward into the movement. The same thing would be done in the Spinal Twist, inhaling to lift the spine and sit up taller and exhaling to rotate deeper into the twist. Once you are holding the position, you can continue to use the breath this way but in a subtler manner. Generally, inhalation is used to lift out of a position and into movements that open, expand, and need strength. Exhalation is used to contract or to stretch and release deeper into postures.

Learn to "move with the breath." This subtle concept involves using the breath to regulate the pace and quality of movements. For example, if you are raising your arms over your head for the Sun Salutation, inhale to lift the chest, shoulders, and arms while keeping your movement and breath timed together. Raise the arms slowly and gracefully and make your inhalation slow and even. Pace breath and movement so that your lungs are full when the movement is complete. When doing a Forward Fold, bend, stretch, and exhale. Continue exhaling while stretching slowly into the pose, finishing the final subtle movements into the stretch at the same time your lungs reach empty. With practice and experimentation, you will understand and master this principle.

You can use your breath to release pain and stiffness. When you have a stiff, tight, or sore area, you can concentrate on your breath and use it to direct energy to the area. Many teachers will say, "Breathe into the painful or tight area." You will find that directing the breath to a location actually works to relax and release it. Using your attention to literally send and feel healing energy and prana move to the place in need relaxes and releases tensions there. This concept is not just a metaphor but a fact, even physically. Oxygen, which is part of the breath, reaches every part of the body. You actually can *breathe into your toes*.

## The Ujjayi Breath

The word *ujjayi* (pronounced oo jaah ee) means "to become victorious" or "to gain mastery," and refers to a special type of breathing used to empower Hatha yoga practice. Ujjayi is done by gently constricting the throat or glottis in order to make a hissing sound. We more or less all know how to do this because it is what we do to give sound to our breath when we whisper. If you say the word "whisper" and prolong the *prrrr* sound, the hissing sound you are making is ujjayi. However, ujjayi is usually done through the nostrils instead of the mouth. The throat is constricted in the same way as is done to whisper, making the same sound on both inhalation and exhalation. To see if you are doing it properly, it is best to be checked by a teacher or experienced student.

When I first began yoga, we learned and used ujjayi only within pranayama breathing practices. We were taught to breathe deeply and evenly or to leave the breath alone during asana practice. I practiced for years this way until I began meeting teachers who emphasized using ujjayi during yoga practice. I experimented for a time with using ujjayi throughout most of my practice and found many positive differences. It improves concentration and endurance while increasing the ability to flow gracefully. Ujjayi improves concentration because it keeps the breath smooth and even. Since this is the breathing pattern that naturally accompanies concentration, it can also be used to aid concentration. With smooth ujjayi, you can become more absorbed in your practice, hold poses longer, effectively regulate heat, and relieve tension. I find using ujjayi in my practice gives an enhanced ability to sense and control energy flows and a general increase in beneficial results.

Some proponents of ujjayi claim it was a long-held secret that unlocks more of the power of asanas. Others advise no control, and argue that the breath should be left free in asana because it will naturally fall into the right groove. Once I was practicing next to a respected Indian yogi who recommends against ujjayi. But he was doing it throughout his practice. When questioned about it, he curtly said, "It is happening naturally because I am doing the poses correctly." However, in my experience, it works both ways. Why wait for the benefits of ujjayi until the postures might correct the breath? Ujjayi brings its own effects and immediate benefits. I recommend experimenting to learn the differences between practicing with and without ujjayi, so that then you will naturally learn how and when to use it. Most students and teachers I suggest this experiment to end up incorporating ujjayi into their practice. This recommendation doesn't imply using ujjayi breath all of the time, but having experimented, you will know its benefits, when to use them, and when to breathe freely. Your breath itself will guide and teach you in myriad ways when you listen to it. Ujjayi can probably be learned from these written instructions, but if you have any doubt, consult a qualified teacher or experienced student. Pranayama, the yogic science of breathing, is also discussed in Chapter 5.

## Toning the Spine

One negative effect of gravity is compression of the spinal column. Spongy, fibrous disks separate the vertebrae of the spine. These disks allow the back to move and they cushion shock and impact. When we sit, stand, or walk, gravity's pull compresses our spinal joints. Many nerve trunks connect the brain and specific body parts or organs through the spinal cord. These nerves exit the spine between the vertebral foramina. When the back is compressed, out of alignment, or if the disks are worn, the nerves can become impinged—cutting the flow of energy and weakening the connecting muscles or organs. A central focus of yoga practice is to maintain or restore suppleness to the spine.

Many yogis measure aging or youthfulness by the flexibility of the spine. I have often seen yogis walking through their classes and pushing on a student's back to test flexibility. When they find an older person with a pliant, limber backbone, they might comment, "Very young man." Conversely, when they see a young but stiff person, they might say, "And here is an old man!" In youth we tend to be flexible and softer, and as we age we tighten and harden—in more ways than just physically. In addition to the effects of gravity, the spine stiffens with age through lack of proper care and use, through injury, and through normal loss of circulation. Our vertebral disks have a venous blood supply until our early twenties. That explains why young people's spines are so resilient and forgiving. By the early twenties the veins that supply the disks have slowly atrophied. Now essential circulation is only obtained through movements of the spine that squeeze and massage nutrients and waste products into and out of the disks. A sedentary person, or even an active person who does not move the entire spine, will slowly lose mobility. Here the saying "use it or lose it" applies clearly.

Hatha yoga focuses a good deal of attention on keeping the spine healthy. The asanas twist or bend the back into every possible position—and even a few of the impossible. These movements keep the disks healthy and pliable. They increase circulation and tone the spine. Many postures work to lengthen the spine and increase spaces between the vertebrae to release nerve impingements. Yoga students also work consciously to hold better posture and to sit erect, which keeps them more alert with more energy flowing to the brain. This generally healthy habit can be overemphasized too. I've seen students become obsessive about keeping the back straight to the point where they seem rigid, mentally and physically. The key is always balance. There is nothing wrong with lounging in a chair or relaxing your posture. When you practice yoga be aware of the effects on the spine. Keep the spine flexible, lengthened, toned, strong, and soft.

## Symmetry and Alignment

The muscular system supports and mobilizes the skeletal structure. Ideally, the muscle sets on both sides of the body would be developed equally to support the body uniformly. Balanced development is especially important along the spinal column where uneven muscle balance can result in misalignment and back problems. Our habits and patterns of movement, however, usually work against maintaining an ideal equilibrium. Most people are right- or left-handed, and most sports are one-sided or unbalanced. For example, golfers and baseball players use either right- or left-handed equipment. Runners often overly tighten the legs, and overwork the lumbar and knees. We usually favor one side of the body when we carry, lift, and exercise. We may also habitually and unconsciously lie, read, or support ourselves more predominantly on one side. In time this tendency overly develops certain muscle sets and creates imbalances in the carriage of the body.

You can try a simple experiment to notice these patterns in your own body. Fold your arms on your chest; then reverse the way you crossed your arms and notice the awkward feeling you get from doing this in an unfamiliar way. Clasp your hands; then change the way you interlocked your fingers and note the feeling. We have become *one-sided*.

The body is also very forgiving and not limited to narrow parameters of alignment. If this were not so we would injure ourselves constantly by poor posture and uncontrolled movement. Asanas are very potent forms. With relatively short holds, of seconds or minutes, asanas can counteract hours of bad posture and misaligned carriage. During asana practice it is important to keep our poses within the range of *structural integrity*—movements that serve and enhance well-being. Learning proper alignment and asana kinesiology while maintaining a softer context that allows some latitude in the way the pose is held is an intelligent approach. Being too rigid about alignment sacrifices flow and grace.

Hatha yoga practice constantly and consciously aims to restore and maintain symmetry and alignment. Practices are designed to work both sides of the body equally, with many postures involving oppositional dynamics. And there is the principle of pose and counterpose in any good sequencing of asanas. Backbends are balanced and complemented by forward bends, and stimulating poses are balanced by tranquilizing poses. Through exploration of well-sequenced poses, the practitioner quickly becomes aware of areas that are misaligned, stiff, weak, or underdeveloped. It is important to become aware of these imbalances and to study changes to the symmetry and alignment in your body when you practice. You can start by observing yourself in a mirror, beginning to notice your body structure. Is one shoulder dropped or lifted? Is there a torque or twist to your frame? Is the pelvis tipped or twisted? Pay attention to particular physical tendencies when you practice the postures and give some extra time to your weaker or stiffer sides in the poses. Students sometimes carelessly do the opposite, once again favoring the stronger or easier direction. Remember, the body's spring tensions have set to hold the body in the positions and attitudes that are habitually held. When you start restructuring and repositioning the body to hold itself in better levels of alignment, you may initially feel awkward and have some resistance from the muscles until the spring dynamics reset to hold at the new levels of balance. Go slowly. Use the postures as tools to restore alignment and start becoming more aware of using your body in more balanced ways during the day. Bring the awareness you develop in yoga to your daily life. Notice when you are holding tension in the muscles. Watch your patterns of sitting, walking, lying, and picking up and carrying things as you move through the day, to see if you can use and balance both sides of the body in ordinary activities. Symmetry of the body is one of the important signs of good health. Asana practice reminds us to look at all sides of things.

## The Three Qualities

Yoga philosophy defines three qualities of nature, called the *three gunas* (goon nah) in Sanskrit. The lowest is *tamas* (pronounced tah muhs), or inertia; the middle is *rajas* (rah juhs), or activity; and the highest is *sattwa* (saht wah), or light. Tamas refers to heaviness, dullness, lethargy, and laziness. Rajas refers to motion, stimulation, intensity, and activity. Sattwa represents clarity, peace, purity, and joy. All things—foods, activities, places, and everything in nature—have one of more of these qualities. We may endeavor to cultivate the higher qualities and higher energies, but the easiest movement is downhill toward tamas, lethargy, or into rajas, activity. It is more difficult to ascend into sattwa, clarity. We tend to stimulate ourselves into activity until we tire ourselves into lethargy, rarely reaching peace and clarity. Knowledge of the three qualities can be applied in an asana practice aimed at balance of the three. All three qualities work together and balance each other. An excess of tamas—or a dull, unconscious practice—results in lethargy and boredom, but in a balanced amount tamas is rest and rejuvenation. Excessive rajas—or an aggressive, overactive practice—can result in nervousness, irritability, or even in tamas. In balance, rajas is energetic and vital. Excessive sattwa, or even too much mental activity, can result in airiness, disorientation, and a lack of grounding, while in balance sattwa brings awareness, peace, and insight. Once again, the three gunas represent a yogic principle that guides us toward achieving balance.

## The Three Root Principles

The triangle is a basic building block in geometry and it is the first stable structure used in construction. A square wall is stabilized by a diagonally placed crossbeam that forms two triangles, adding strength and structure. In the same way, using the Three Root Principles strengthens your foundation in yoga. In the *chakra* system (to be explained in detail later), the root chakra resides at the base of the spine. Inside the symbol for this center is an upside-down triangle. The placement of this basic geometric figure symbolizes both the mystical aspects of the sacrum, which is also an inverted triangle, and also the three principles of *iccha, kriya,* and *jnana* (pronounced itch uh, kree yuh, and nyaah nuh, as in mañana).

Iccha signifies will power or intention; kriya means the power of action or technique; and jnana refers to the power of knowledge. By using all three of these powers we form a triangle in our practice that is a stronger and more effective structure than we could build from any one principle alone. When performing any asana or pranayama, the benefits are increased by using and executing the proper form and technique (kriya), having knowledge about the technique and its function (jnana), and, finally, by using our will and focused intention (iccha) to enhance and direct the desired effects. Maintaining a balance of these principles becomes another form of conscious practice wherein we seek to stay present while directing the form and energy of the asana or pranayama.

## Relaxation

Modern life has unfortunately made scarcities of peace and freedom from tension. Many people come to yoga solely for its tension-relieving qualities. Stress is a major factor in aging and the degeneration of health. It has also been shown to cause dysfunction of the immune system and cancer. The body and mind need regular rest and relaxation, but true relaxation is more than merely resting. True relaxation involves balancing and restoring energies. Yoga excels in providing rejuvenating relaxation. Deep relaxation and restoration of equilibrium require the release of pent-up energy and stored blocks. Yoga asanas and breathing circulate life force and release blockages.

Physical memories of emotional experiences and psychological trauma can be stored in the musculature. Our instincts cause us to tense our necks and hunch forward when fearful or frightened in order to protect our vital organs. Emotions affect the body and organs in myriad ways. The circulatory effects, deep stretching, and energetic releases experienced with asana practice can remove old, stored emotional blocks. Students very often experience an emotional and psychological catharsis from the postures. During practice it is not uncommon for someone actually to experience a release of pent-up anger or fear or to recall the experience that caused it. This process is an important factor in stress relief, whether or not we are conscious of our accumulated tensions. Even the small irritations we endure each day can cause neck, chest, or low back tensions that should be relieved each day.

A simple experiment can demonstrate how storing tension affects consciousness. Tense your neck slightly while pushing your chin about an inch forward. Notice how this makes you feel. Hold that position for a few moments as though that tightness was permanently in your neck. When you release this position, you should notice a great relief. More profound shifts in attitude can be experienced when deeper, more unconsciously held tensions are eliminated.

Relaxation balances activity and activity balances relaxation. Each creates a need for the other. I advise regularly taking a day off each week from your practice. This day off can be a fixed day of the week or a "circumstantial" day—when situation or obligation prevents practice. I know teachers who claim to practice every day without a rest for any reason. Rest is part of balanced living and a weekly day of rest is found in traditions all over the world. It is also important to have a period of rest after your practice session. The final posture in every practice session should be *Savasana*, the Corpse pose. What is more relaxed than a corpse? Savasana implies a special quality of conscious relaxation and the separation of awareness from the outer body. "Getting out of the way" by withdrawing from external awareness allows one's inner somatic intelligence to put things in order. This self-directed process is very effective in restoring balance and energy in a short period of time. It may be very tempting to skip over Savasana but it is important to include it. Practice should be a means of self-healing. If we think of asana practice as a kind of *self-surgery*, final relaxation in Savasana is analogous to going into the recovery room after an operation to allow energy to circulate and the body to heal and balance itself.

## Flow and Grace

As we progress in asana practice, it is very beneficial to develop qualities of grace and flow in moving between the poses. In the same way that we compartmentalize our lives, we may tend to fragment our practice into a series of syncopated movements. We may focus on the goal of reaching the posture we are moving toward and pay less attention to interesting processes of transition. This static focus leads to mechanical movements and less graceful practice. You can bring a gracefulness and fluidity to your movements by making the journey between postures as important as the destination of the finished pose.

In addition to moving smoothly with a dance-like flow, there is another, more elusive, quality to discover and develop in the poses and through the transitions between them. I call it *laghima,* a Sanskrit word meaning to float or levitate. Great dancers or athletes seem to glide and float effortlessly through their movements. They have worked hard to attain their performance levels, but they are no longer forcing it. They are moving in grace and joy. Laghima is a combination of strength, flexibility, flow, and balance. It may be difficult to describe, but we have all seen it and any of us can learn it. This lightness and floating sensation also relates to balancing the flows of upward and downward moving energies, and the relationship of control and surrender described in the next chapter. Even a beginner can start learning to flow gracefully through the practice. Remember, Siva, the mythological first yogi, was also the great dancer. By learning to dance through our practice, we will find more benefit and more joy.

## Personal Practice

There are many ways to learn yoga—studying from books, teachers, fellow students, taking classes, or using the many videos available today. However you learn, it is important to develop a personal practice you do yourself. One of the great things about yoga is that it can be done almost anywhere, with little space and with no special tools or equipment. Some unique learning possibilities and qualities of experience can only happen when practicing solo. You can learn to follow your own flow of energy and to tune into your specific needs for that moment. Practicing alone can make it easier to get into a deeper inner space, communion, and personal flow. As you advance in your ability to maintain a personal practice, a special quality of experience can also develop. The innate intelligence of the body actually begins to guide the practice and an inner-directed process that can be very healing and nurturing begins to unfold.

Group practice also offers particular advantages for learning and can be very valuable. We receive a lot of energy and inspiration when practicing with others. Group practice is synergistic—each participant seems to get more out of the class than he or she puts in. When practicing with a group or leader, however, it is harder to synchronize with and create your own inner flow as well as you can when working independently. Many students become so dependent on external supports for their practice that they cannot practice or continue on their own when necessary. For teachers, the strength of teaching is intimately related to the strength of personal practice. For these reasons I recommend that serious students—and certainly yoga teachers—benefit from their own personal sessions regularly. If you have the opportunity to take classes consistently, you may only work alone on occasion, but it is important to do so. Personal practice will lead to many discoveries, to self-reliance, and your yoga will develop its own momentum.

When you approach yoga practice as a personal process of learning to listen, to work with, and respond to your own inner feedback systems, you become your own teacher. Discoveries unique to your body and your own special energy are available to you alone. Instead of just learning a particular series of selected poses, you develop a process of constant discovery that continues to grow and evolve. Personal practice may stay the same for a period of time, then it may change occasionally or more frequently during different periods of life. The varying circumstances of each day affects your needs and your practice. The context of yoga is your whole daily life and an entire lifetime, and in this context of practice grows and changes with you as you move through the circle of life. This broad context includes everything you are doing, and not doing, with your body, and how all these things affect you physically. Learn to use yoga to tune yourself physically and to balance all of the things you do.

Yoga practice complements and balances all other activities, and inactivity, as well as providing the very unique benefits of Hatha yoga.

Walking, hiking, athletics, long sitting, rest, and sleep are all part of the mix and part of the whole life context you work with in your personal practice. Looking upon your personal practice as continuously discovering and rediscovering, honing and fine tuning makes it your own unique yoga, specifically for yourself. Personal practice is a well to draw from; it is one of the greatest gifts we can give ourselves, and it is ultimately a gift to others too.

## Integrating Yoga into Daily Life

There are numerous ways to integrate yogic practices into the day. Many techniques in the tradition were gleaned from watching animals. An animal will stretch several times a day to relieve the stiffness from inactivity. Humans, on the other hand, tend to compartmentalize life. If our workout class is at five, we may be sedentary the rest of the day and not give exercise a thought. Many people will even circle around and around the parking lot looking for a space a hundred feet closer to the door of the gym they are going to work out in.

Look for opportunities to walk, and walk briskly, or use the stairs when possible. In order to stay flexible, get in the practice of stretching out stiffness after sitting for long periods. A simple standing forward bend, a back arch, and twist will make a real difference. Stand up, breathe, and move around at regular intervals to break up long sedentary periods. Create your own "chair yoga" by learning to do twists and forward bends occasionally at your desk or in the car. Sit a good portion of the time with a straight spine and practice walking some of the time with alignment and awareness. Watch how you carry things. When picking things up, consciously use the alignment you learn from your yoga practice and make a forward bend asana out of the movement. Start using both sides of your body evenly. If, for example, you are leaning or reading on one side for a time, balance yourself by switching to the other side. Your yoga practice will also make you more aware of your tendencies to hold tension. Do you tense your neck when you write, type, or even when you watch movies or television? Try using some of your television time to do some easy stretches or passive asanas while watching. Become more attentive during the day so that you notice and eliminate bad postural habits. You should also be mindful not to get carried away by all this self-observation—a little bit goes a long way. You do not want to be constantly controlled or contrived in your actions; you just want to be aware and occasionally restore balance. It is more important in the long run to be relaxed and spontaneous than to be overly self-conscious and controlled.

The other day a few friends and I had the chance to visit a great museum. One member of our group was an avid, perhaps fanatic, yoga practitioner. Even though he had been regularly practicing for many days, he said he could not go with us because he would miss his morning practice. He reminded me of the friend described earlier who wouldn't go on the city and river tour with us. I told him that one of the reasons I practice yoga is to enjoy life; I suggested that we could go, but not miss our practice, finding a way to work it in. As we walked for hours touring the museum and grounds, we found a way to inconspicuously do many postures and stretches. We used railings to do twists and forward bends and did some squat poses to release tension accumulating in our legs and lower backs. We even did a couple of partner poses. All this was woven right into our day. That night we felt the glow of a good physical workout and spirits lifted by art, conversation, and insights. My legs were a bit sore from climbing and walking so much, so before bed I used about ten minutes of forward bending and lunges to release the tightness. My friend was happy he had changed his routine. This is another example of how yoga can be incorporated during daily activities and how it complements our lives without taking out time or preventing us from our activities.

We weaken our backs by habitually reclining on chairs and couches. It is invaluable to learn to sit on the floor without support. When you first start, simple sitting can be difficult and uncomfortable but staying with it will increase flexibility and the tone of back muscles. I was once spending a weekend at the home of a friend and former yoga teacher. He hadn't practiced in several years and had gotten stiff and paunchy. I happened to be sitting with my feet crossed in the Lotus posture, talking to my friend who slouched on a couch. He was explaining that he no longer had time to keep up his practice. I realized that I was actually doing yoga while we spoke, by sitting in the Lotus pose, and I pointed that out. I told him about an old text I had read that said one could get many of the benefits of practice simply by sitting for a time each day in the Lotus pose. When I first read it I thought it was just glorifying the benefits of that famous asana, but later I realized that it was true. Sitting on the floor in any cross-legged pose brings flexibility to the hips, legs, and ankles while toning the spine and creating a flow of energy throughout the whole body. No matter how busy we are, we can find time to sit on the floor. Many yogis even enjoy sitting cross-legged in chairs. When done properly, sitting this way can actually be more comfortable and better for circulation.

At the end of the day, before bed, it's a good idea to spend a few minutes for an evening rebalancing and unwinding. Do some forward bends, twists, or stretches to relieve any tightness or tension in the body. A relaxed Shoulderstand can also be very helpful at the end of the day, too. There is great benefit to completing the day this way and it doesn't take much time. Even a few minutes of calming poses will bring hours of better sleep and help to maintain overall flexibility and energy from day to day. As you begin to bring awareness of your body's energies into daily life, you will find many ways to incorporate the benefits of yoga into the day without taking any extra time. In fact, it will add much time and energy to your days. In the same way, many of the principles explained in this chapter can be applied to other areas of living. Then all daily activities and the insights gained from them can contribute to yogic practice and to general well-being. This awareness and these mini practices may take a bit more energy in the moment but will reward you with much more strength and energy in the long run.

## Enjoying Your Practice

In the section on discipline we discussed the importance of learning to enjoy one's practice. As a teacher I've noticed that students who enjoy their yoga are the ones who stay with it over the long term. Some people make their practice, if not their lives, a constant struggle. They seem to be always pushing their limits, working on their form, or weighing and measuring themselves—trying to get to *where they should be*. Their approach becomes forced and tense. It has served me to approach yoga more softly—to learn to enjoy it. We need to work hard and with discipline, but we also have to lighten up and remove the tendency toward regimentation. I recommend, even to my newest students, that everyone spend some of their practice time working at a level they can enjoy and that they regularly stay within their level of enjoyment for entire sessions. Even for a beginner with limited abilities, there is an enjoyable level of practice. I have taught more than one person in a wheelchair who discovered more joy of movement than many of us may ever find.

We can also work hard and still stay within enjoyment. We can all push the envelope and work near our maximum edges. Certainly we need to make special efforts at times in order to make progress, but if we always struggle to do our utmost, we lose energy and tire.

We all have a range of movement where we must exert and another range where we can move more freely. I recommend practicing in the latter at least as often as the former. We can find that range of movement where we feel good, flowing in the joy of exercise and motion, and visit it often. We can learn to use yoga to get into higher, elevated states, making it fun, enjoyable. It's a great secret for maintaining a lifelong practice of yoga.

CHAPTER 5

# The Internal Alchemy of Hatha Yoga

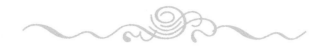

Along with the physical, Hatha yoga involves mental and internal processes of development. As one progresses through the asanas, the inner process takes on more importance and moves the practice to subtler levels that yield benefits in many areas of living. Learning about and bringing attention to the inner dynamics in asana will open new dimensions and possibilities in practice. Over time, cultivating an inner focus will make our physical practices far more interesting, engaging, and effective. There is literally no end to the exploration of the psychophysical organism.

When we begin the practice of Hatha yoga, we primarily focus on the more obvious challenges posed by the physical movements. New students commonly ask, "How can I become more flexible?" "What do I need to do in order to twist into that pose?" Or, "Will I ever be able to do the Headstand?" As we gain more mastery of alignment and structures in asanas, we turn our attention toward the poses' subtler aspects—toward the movement of internal energy and the inner dynamics. Alchemy, a magical process of transmutation of the mundane into the precious, originated in the search for ways to change base metals into gold. This search for material transformations was the beginning of modern chemistry, but alchemists also pursued a more secret and inner quest in the search for an elixir of longevity. In this chapter, as in Chapter 4, we explore the interplay and interaction of physical, mental, and spiritual components in yoga that help us in the magical, alchemical transmutation of our practice from common physical exercise into radiant health, awareness, and longevity.

## The Dance of Energy

Science has shown dramatically how energy and matter are part of a single spectrum. The two, like particles and waves, are, in fact, one relationship—what modern physicists call a "field." All of life can be seen as a dance of the universal energy field. Hatha, the yoga of balancing sun and moon polarities, has its foundation in this transformative dance. The mythological source of this yoga of transformation is the god Siva, who is symbolized as the great dancer, dancing in a ring of fire. This image of a dancing divinity implies the cosmic dance of energy, birth, death, and transformation. Everything that enters fire is changed. Learning about the movement and flow of energy is one of the core principles of Hatha yoga.

### The Energy Body

In yoga practice we can experience both physical and nonphysical forms of energy. Physical forms also include many energetic fields—metabolic, electromagnetic, gravitational, thermal. Nonphysical energy forms include the movement of prana, or life force, healing energy, feelings of well-being, and the flow of consciousness, attention, and awareness. In the Triangle pose, for example, electrical currents and consciousness flow back and forth between the brain and muscles throughout the body. A lifting feeling comes from pressing the feet into the ground and an equal and opposite descending feeling meets it. A sense of well-being and pranic energy can be made to flow in the body and there is mental concentration moving to different points while attention sees all parts of the body simultaneously. All of this can be referred to as awareness of the energy body. Becoming aware of the energy body in all postures is the beginning of cultivating the inner practice of yoga.

Every posture has important principles of structure, alignment, and kinesiology, but equally important to these mechanical aspects of asana is learning about the internal movements of energy. Muscles and bones are articulated and activated by flows of energy. Our practice can be broadened and deepened by expanding it beyond attention only to external form and including awareness and emphasis on the quality of energy and feeling in the postures. It is not only how far we move into a given posture that matters, but also improving the quality of the flow of energies. Energy flows can be strengthened, made more dynamic; energy currents through the nerves can be increased, and healing qualities improved. All of these dynamics and benefits make yoga more effective and enjoyable.

I was watching a friend do some yoga informally while watching TV. I saw her struggling farther into the Forward Fold pose. I came over and offered to share an insight with her. She immediately said, "No, no, it will hurt, I'm stiff, I can't go any farther!" I told her my suggestion wasn't about going farther into her edges, but about developing a deeper inner quality. She tensed and said she was already doing all she could. I noticed her resistance and fear and just asked her to back off in the pose, not to stretch as far. She was trying to grab her toes, and I suggested she grab her ankles instead. Once she was no longer struggling, I was able to have her lift her chest, extend her torso, and drop her shoulders to release tension in the neck area. Through acknowledging her fear and resistance, I guided her into a variation of the posture wherein she could feel good energy flow in her legs and along her spine, and where she could experience a general sense of well-being in the posture. This was the first time she had done an asana that way. She had thought she always had to go to her maximum, pushing her maximum edge. It can be beneficial to push to a maximum edge or limit of flexibility or strength at times, but it is equally important, if not more important, also to have regular practice in an enjoyable range of movement and ability that focuses on better feelings and internal energy flows. Both approaches to asanas are useful and have different ends.

## Upward and Downward Energy

The body has two principle directions of energy, upward moving energy and downward moving energy. In youth, upward moving energy is rising and at its peak, like plants growing and rising toward the sun. Children seem to have an endless supply. They are always in movement, at times almost "bouncing off the walls," and we often advise them to "settle down." Children are hard to keep down, while the aged are hard to get up. Throughout youth we are growing taller, lifting and expanding. Ideally in adulthood the two energies are balanced. But, as we age, upward moving energy begins to decrease and we're more affected by the downward pull of gravity. Our bodies begin to shrink, sag, hunch over, and stoop down. In the womb we are like a seed; our body is in the embryo position waiting to grow and expand, and then outwardly blossoming throughout the period of youth. As we become older our bodies tend to fold and shrink inwardly back toward the womb. Many of our elders are no longer able to stand erect. They bend at the knees and waist and have curved upper spines, often needing a cane to walk. The aging body folds back toward the embryo position. These patterns can be changed, or at least greatly slowed down, with yoga.

Upward moving energy should be cultivated and consciously strengthened during practice. Downward moving energy, aided by gravity, tends to take care of itself. Gravity is essentially a compressional field. Our bodies are being pulled down, or compressed, by gravity, and the structure of our physical bodies has evolved to lift and extend against gravity. Many asanas create an extensional field of energy and movement that works in opposition to, and in concert with, gravity. Gravity is a major factor in aging and the slumping and sagging of the body, but it is not our enemy. We have discussed how our dependence on gravity has been demonstrated by some of the physical problems astronauts must deal with in a weightless environment. Through prolonged periods of weightlessness, their muscles would atrophy and their bones would decalcify unless they work out with springs and isometric tensions. Our bodies require a dynamic field to work against and take root into in order to function properly. Gravity is our friend.

A simple experiment will show you how to begin to become aware of how you function in the gravitational field and how upward and downward forces work together. Come into a basic standing position with feet parallel and a couple of inches apart. Slightly bend the knees and slightly curve your spine forward, allowing the shoulders to stoop and the neck to bend. Take notice of how you feel and of the increase in the downward pull; also take careful notice of the change in consciousness. Now begin pressing your feet down into the floor. This *pressing* is actually a lifting of muscular energy created biomechanically. Use this lifting feeling to straighten the knees and continue bringing this lift up through the hips and spine until you are standing as tall as possible. Finally, lift your chest and let the shoulders roll backward. Again, notice the difference in consciousness and in how you feel. Hold this standing position and continue pressing your feet down to increase the upward flow of energy. Even if you stop pressing the feet you should still be able to feel the upward flow.

As an additional experiment, add Mula Bandha, the contraction and lifting of the anal sphincter muscles, to the pose. See if you can notice the difference in the upward energy. Now add conscious breathing. When you inhale, feel the lifting; when you exhale, maintain the lift while allowing energy to circulate. Using ujjayi breathing will further increase the effects. These techniques can be applied in the practice of many of the asanas. Holding this standing position statically while creating an inner, upward flow of energy creates what I call a "standing wave" in the body.

**Standing Waves**

Standing waves are an underlying dynamic structural pattern in the universe. Standing waves are nontraveling waves of energy or vibration that maintain fixed wavelengths and frequency. In other words, they have lots of energy moving through them but they look like they are standing still. When a river drops over an irregularity in its bed, or over a large rock, a standing wave develops with its curl facing upstream. This standing wave will look like a large mound of water and appear to be relatively still and stable, but the river is literally pouring through it. When a strong wind lifts over a mountain top, a standing wave in the air flow develops across the peak, often expressed as an elliptical shaped cloud.

Asanas themselves actually are, in a sense, standing waves. Energy can flow dynamically within the body even as a pose is held statically. Standing waves appear to be still but have constant movement within them. Standing waves demonstrate a delicate interplay of static and dynamic opposites balanced in time. An ancient yogic text states, "A yogi is one who sees movement in stillness, and stillness in movement." Generating and riding standing waves and *surfing* internal waves of energy in asana practice is one way to experience this. There is the stillness of asana with the internal dynamic movement of energy. This is contrasted by the stillness of attention and awareness within the dynamic movement of asana and energy. Physical standing waves can be created by balancing opposing, internal tensions and by bringing equilibrium to the interplay of strength and flexibility. They create feelings of inner power and well-being, bringing a sense of wholeness to the posture. Discovering this is a revelation and brings a forward leap in one's practice.

**Lines of Energy**

The concept of lines of energy refers to the intentional creation of energy flows along channels or directions in the body. Working with and developing lines of energy in yoga poses refines and increases the benefits of the poses. Yogi Joel Kramer, who articulated this concept, defines it as follows: "Lines of energy are vibratory currents that move in different directions within each posture. The intensity of these currents in the nerves can be controlled by the muscles and has a feeling that moves in an outward direction."

You can easily experience this directional energy flow by coming again to a standing position. Raise your arms directly out to your sides, parallel to the floor. Extend and lengthen the arms outward, toward the side walls of the room. You can now experience the extensional feeling from the lines of energy moving along the arms. This flow can be increased by making sure your arms are extending all the way to the ends of the fingers, and even beyond to the walls, without breaking or bending at the joints. This extensional movement energizes and brings vibrancy to the arms, but it also opens the neck and shoulders. Next, begin pressing the feet until you feel lines of energy moving down into and coming up from the floor. Try to allow this flow from the floor to connect with and move out through the flow along the arms. Connecting and linking the various energy flows creates more beneficial effects and structural integrity in the postures. All postures have these lines and flows to be discovered and worked with. Don't increase the flow to a point of tension, overexertion, or contraction. The energy lines will help you align and adjust your postures because when the flow feels good and moves freely internally, the posture is usually properly aligned.

In addition to moving particular lines of energy through the limbs and torso, you also want to experience a general feeling of movement of the entire energy body. In a twisting pose, for example, the energy body itself feels like it is twisting. In a backbend it feels like it is arching back. Often when students see themselves with video or photographic feedback, they are surprised that they feel like they are bending farther than the picture shows. This is usually because they feel the movement of the energy body more than the physical body actually moving. I discovered this difference once when having an instant photo made of an asana I was doing. I wanted to see how far back I was bending and had a friend take my photo. I felt like I was bending much farther than the actual pose shown in the picture. With some experimentation I realized that my energy body was bending much more than the physical body. It is good to be able to sense this non-physical movement and to use and accentuate it in postures. Whether or not you are able to move fully into a pose physically, you can still move the corresponding internal energy. This inner movement actually creates and maintains physical structure and support and, in time, you will be able to move into a fuller pose. Actually all physical movements are preceded and controlled by this flow of energy.

Keeping your energy active makes the body radiant and vibrant in the postures and prolongs youthfulness. The awareness and posture you cultivate will carry over from yoga practice to daily life. We eventually learn to walk taller, keep our spines supple and straight, and keep our energy channels open throughout the day. The effects of gravity and aging are balanced and our vitality increases. Lifting your energy up will help to uplift you too. Smiling lifts the spirit and is an indicator that your energy is flowing upward. One of the goals of yoga is the alchemical transformation from being down, heavy, sad, and lethargic to being up, happy, high, energetic, and clear.

## Withdrawing Energy

We concentrate more often on creating and extending energy into parts of the body. Learning to withdraw energy is the other, equally important, side of this coin. You can learn to pull energy out of a limb or body part. When you do a pose more passively, energy is withdrawn and the limb is moved or stretched. For example, in a forward bend, instead of energizing the leg muscles they can be made passive, the energy withdrawn, and then the muscles are stretched by using leverage from the arms and weight from the trunk. Savasana, the Corpse pose, is the ulti-mate in energy withdrawal. You learn and develop the ability to con-sciously withdraw your energy body and your conscious awareness from all parts of the body. This total withdrawal happens naturally in sleep, of course, but in Savasana it is a cultivated ability that, once learned, permits you to recharge and renew your energetic and physi-cal bodies in a very short period of time.

**Mental Energy**

Understanding the dance of energy includes becoming sensitive and aware of how certain patterns of thought, feeling, and mental energy can lift you up or pull you down, lowering your life force into weak-ness, lethargy, and even illness. By seeing downward tendencies when they rise in predominance in yourself, you can learn to generate the inner positive thought force to transform them into upward moving energy. This transformation must be in balance, allowing natural rhythms of relaxation, passivity, and inactivity to flow through their normal cycles in daily life. One simple measure of upward or down-ward moving psychological energy is the smile and frown. Smiles, of course, raise our energy and vibration. We could all learn to use the benefits of smiling more often.

## Aligning and Adjusting Asanas from Within and Without

Learning how to align postures properly for your particular body, age, and stage of development is another example of learning to balance internal and external information systems. By external information, I refer to the way asanas are shown in books, by teachers, in photo-graphs, and in classes. These are not always just idealized postures but often represent what a particular school, lineage, or teacher feels is the correct way to do specific asanas. Of course, there are differing, sometimes opposing, opinions among various lineages and schools. Internal information refers to the immediate feedback of information and effects that a pose gives you during your own practice. Both external and internal information should play important roles in guiding your practice.

As we have discussed, Hatha yoga developed from inspiration, experimentation, watching animals, and the discovery of structural, archetypal movements inherent in the body. All these sources have formed a body of information and tradition that we now draw from in our study of yoga. Whether or not one puts great faith in tradition, we have seen that there is no one yoga approach and that opinions differ about even the most basic alignments of particular asanas. How, then, is one to find one's way?

An essential part of learning how to find the right asanas, practices, and alignments is learning to listen to the effects—hear the feedback from your body, and develop your awareness of how the postures affect you in the moment and over time. This development of internal awareness and attunement is balanced and enhanced by external knowledge and information. Some people try to delineate which postures are appropriate for different body types, constitutions, times of year, for males, females, certain age groups, and so on. While this information may be useful, theoretically, and possibly accurate, it must be balanced by developing the ability to respond internally to your actual practice with all your capacities and all your senses. Using both internal and external information systems, you can circumvent practicing solely by technique and belief and, instead, learn and develop from your own direct experience and perception. The internal and external offer two differing vantage points that balance and guide each other. Sometimes holding a posture in a particular form can feel good, but a book or teacher might show you that you are not holding the pose in a beneficial way. You may have become accustomed to an improperly aligned position and it began to feel good. External feedback from another person, or even a mirror, can help improve your pose and correct your inner guidance system. Similarly, holding a beneficial alignment sometimes doesn't feel as good as the incorrect alignment until the body is brought into balance. Either internal or external information is sometimes incorrect, but using and developing awareness of how both perspectives balance each other will guide your practice.

A posture I use to exemplify this is the Extended Warrior pose, *Parsvakonasana*. You will be able to follow the theory given here even if you are not familiar with this posture. The Extended Warrior is the standing pose done in a single plane with the back leg kept straight, the front shin at a right angle to the floor, and torso extended out over the front leg, weight on the lower arm through the hand on the floor. There are differing opinions among leading teachers about where the front hand and arm should be. Many books and teachers show the front hand placed on the floor along the outside edge of the front foot; others teach the hand being moved to the floor along the inside of the front foot arch. As an additional variation, the front arm can be bent supporting the trunk with the forearm placed on the thigh, but many teachers object to this adaptation, saying it compromises the classical position. Guidance can be found in listening to the effects of the pose.

Two of the purposes of this Warrior pose are toning and strengthening the whole body, and improving concentration and attention. Different front hand or arm placements have little to no effect on these aspects of the posture. Similarly, different front hand or arm positions have little effect on the flexibility-building aspects of this pose. But another key benefit of this position is relieving tension and compression in the lumbar spine, and hand placement has a big effect here. As one extends forward into the posture, the torso is rolled open while the chest is lifted. This twisting, opening extension relieves tightness and pressure in the lumbar. Moving the hand position to the inside of the foot frees the torso to twist and open more. I have experimented with many students and body types in this pose and find very few who can place their hand in the accepted position, to the outside of the foot, and get as many beneficial effects, as they do when placing their hand by the inside of the foot—yet many teachers still say this placement is not correct. Furthermore, by bending the arm and supporting their torso on the thigh, the majority of students are able to get even more opening and benefit while sacrificing nothing—it is an improvement, not a compromise. When you tune into the effects of the pose as you experiment with the different hand placements, you will notice which modification gives you the most freedom, opening, the best flow of energy, and sense of well-being. I use this example to show how we can use traditional information about the poses but also need to listen within to guide and move our postures to the optimal position for our individual needs and abilities.

In earlier stages of practice, perhaps for several years, it is important to follow predominantly the teachings, practices, and techniques learned from qualified sources. During this time you should allow your own unique inner process to awaken and develop, and look for teachers who encourage this personal development. This inner process can develop from the beginning, even while you follow instructions and practices from a teacher. While learning, you emphasize receiving information, and as you progress you put more emphasis on your own inner process. Don't focus only on getting into the posture, but consider also what you are getting out of each posture. *Form follows function;* this principle of design can also be applied to asana. The form of the asana is secondary to the desired effects it produces. Adjust poses by using the alignment that creates the best energy flow, by means of internal feedback and internal effects of the pose. When you are not sure of how to align an asana, pay attention to what others have said and also to which modifications give you the best results and best flow of energy. This is the bottom line—not a picture in a book or a teacher's assertions, but what your body is telling you. Making sense out of conflicting opinions about asana practice involves balancing what you have learned from others with your own experience and inner guidance.

## Surfing the Edges

Every yoga posture has different levels and intensities of engagement, and every body has its own limits. You can learn to adjust and modulate these levels, or *edges,* in order to get different effects and benefits out of the asanas. This technique was also pioneered in yoga in the sixties by Joel Kramer, who called it "playing the edges." I use the term "surfing" because it implies flow, balance, adjustment, and enjoyment—while riding on a wave of energy. Learning to surf and to experiment with the many different types of edges can add beneficial dimensions of subtlety to your practice.

Some useful edges to learn and be attentive to are edges of strength, flexibility, balance, endurance, fear, and pain. The concept of working with edges is taking hold in yoga, but it is often presented in a limited manner that misses the subtlety and sophistication of this process. The concept is not limited to the idea of "staying on your edge," or working near your maximum. Instead, it embraces an entire arena involving working with many different types of edges and many different levels for each type of edge. Surfing the edges does not only refer to "pushing the envelope" or working near your maximum limits of possibility, but includes riding the waves, understanding and using the whole range of levels within your ability for various effects and benefits.

Flexibility is a good place to begin to learn how to work with your edges. The measurement of the edge is noticed at the minimum and, more important, the maximum limit. As you begin to move into a posture, the place where you start to meet the first sensations or feelings of resistance and stiffness is called the minimum edge. The maximum edge is the point where you feel you can move no further into the posture without pain or injury. The intermediate edge is halfway between these two points.

Edges of strength are defined in the same way or can often be noticed by increasing strain, "efforting," or shaking. These are important demarcations of beginning, intermediate, and maximum edges of flexibility. Working with edges is like using a volume control in your practice to adjust the intensity and level of the postures. You can learn the differences between practicing at minimum edges, maximum edges, and varying points in between, simply by beginning to use these levels. Experiment with them and watch how the different levels affect the alignment of your poses and the inner experience of your practice. Once you get the sense of surfing edges in one area of your practice, it is easy to learn in others.

Remember, working at the maximum edges can be exhilarating, but always working at the maximum edges of strength and flexibility can become frustrating, exhausting, and possibly lead to injury. Backing off and working at a 75-percent edge can increase the level of enjoyment—another important edge. Backing off to intermediate edges, even in simple poses, can allow work in other areas such as alignment or endurance, or exploration of the counterplay of isometric and isotonic pressures—pressing externally and resisting internally to change effects of the posture, explained in a later section. (Using pain as an edge and teacher for healing is more complicated and will be explained in Chapter 7.)

Find your edges by beginning to move and then noticing the sensations. Stay well short of the maximum edges until your body is warmed up. You may sometimes be able to bend completely in half, for example, but your maximum edges of resistance will come well before that until you are warm and have good circulation. Let's say you are starting with a series of Sun Salutations. Don't begin with your best, most technically perfect poses. Don't start at your maximum edges. Instead, warm up and slowly approach your maximum edges with successive repetitions of the salutations. This actually makes warming up easier and you will have less muscle soreness and much less risk of injury. It is like recapitulating the steps through which you progressed and learned from the beginning.

Each time you begin your practice, pay particular attention to where your edges are that day. Edges are on the move constantly, day to day and breath to breath. Where you work in relation to these edges will have a large impact on the quality and result of your practice. Every day you have a different body. The time of day you begin, the foods you have eaten, and your activities the previous day all have a big effect. By watching these relationships you will learn a lot. Your own body and your own practice will teach you how to surf the edges.

## Flow, the Dance of Control and Surrender

Hatha yoga has a close relationship with Raja yoga, the eight-limbed path we have already discussed. The third and fourth limbs of this eightfold path are asana and pranayama—posture and breath. One of the core principles of Raja yoga is control. This system seeks mastery in living through a refined ability to control the mind, body, senses, breath, and consciousness itself. We need not look far, however, to see that there are vast areas beyond our control. In fact, we are able to control only a very small arena in our lives. Beyond control, we must also learn to surrender and dance in harmony with the many crosscurrents of life in which we find ourselves. Watching and learning from the interplay of control and surrender in asana is an important dimension to include in one's practice.

This insight was brought home to me while swimming in the rapids of a river in California. It was a beautiful summer afternoon and I was sunning on a large rock next to the river and watching some fish swimming. I decided to join them and jumped in the river. I first swam upstream against the swift current. After using up a lot of energy and making little progress, I tired and started swimming downstream, carried by the current. I decided to relax completely, to surrender to current and let it take me. It wasn't long till I was nearly crashed on some rocks. So I started controlling and swimming strongly, but again this was crashing me into the rocks. Soon I discovered what the fish were doing. I found an exhilarating balance of control and surrender, constantly adjusting my efforts on this interface so that I could jet down the river, riding the current and darting around the boulders. I then turned upstream and experimented swimming in different intensities of the current and finding eddies to help me travel back up to my starting point. I spent the afternoon playing on this edge of control and surrender and the lessons learned changed my yoga practice, even my life.

Great athletes and great dancers seem to glide effortlessly through their movements. We know how much work and effort they must have gone through to reach the place of flowing in effortlessness. To become a great runner, swimmer, dancer, or yogi, we must cross the threshold between the mechanical action of effort to the realm of flow and grace. We must first learn the mechanical movements, then later let go of them. At the level of flow, the body seems to move freely and gracefully by itself, out of its own intelligence. The flow itself dances, swims, or does yoga.

We often start out in a new physical endeavor with struggle, strain, awkwardness, and tightness—we are fighting to gain and learn control. When we reach a level of mastery and effortless flow, it is no longer control or surrender, but the birth of a new expression born of these two. Flow is an interplay of pushing through and backing off, of holding on and letting go, of upward moving energy and downward moving energy, and of structure and free form. When all of these polarities come into play, they yield a fruit that is beyond any one of them. The word Hatha points to these poles. *Ha* reminds us of the sun, of structure and control. *Tha* reminds us to let go, back off, to surrender. How do we attain the balance of the two? It is not attained; rather, it is discovered. If we explain in too much detail about how to attain a balance of control and surrender, it eludes us and becomes only control. If we surrender too much trying to give up control, we are dashed on the rocks. I learned this lesson the hard way in the mountains. I was skiing down a steeper hill than I usually attempted, behind a friend who was an Olympic skier. He suggested I follow him and glean something from his movements. He seemed to float gracefully, effortlessly down the hill, dancing from side to side. I followed him and picked it up, flowing and dancing my way behind him. Then I thought, "Great, now I know how to do this, I just balance control and surrender!" But when I started to think and analyze, I had moved out of the flow and back in to the rigidity of control. The next thing I knew I was flying through the air and I landed on my head, my body in a knot. Fortunately, I had done yoga that day and didn't get injured like I might have had I been too stiff or tight. My body said, "I'm glad that I've been in this position before." We can learn about the interplay of control and surrender in asana by experimenting with pushing through and letting go, with tightening and softening, holding poses dynamically and actively, or passively. We can emphasize the control side of the equation by strengthening the lines of energy, actively holding the pose and working nearer our maximum edges. This emphasis will tone and energize the body. Practicing on the surrender side of the equation, we can soften, let go, and let gravity do the work, easing our emphasis on alignment and letting the stretch go deeper into the muscles. Become aware of these polarities and the dance will lead to their marriage and the fruit of joy, flow, and grace.

## Pranayama—The Mastery of Energy

The word *pranayama* is usually translated as breath control. *Prana* means "to breathe forth" and it also refers to life force or the energy of life. *Yama* means to restrain or control. The yamas are the restraints and controls in the first limb of Patanjali's yoga and Yama, curiously, is also the name of the god of death. Pranayama is the study of our breath and life force. Yogis have pointed out that, although we feel like separate individuals, we are not as separate as we feel. Our continuous inhalations and exhalations remind us that we are interdependent on and interconnected with all things—with the matrix of life. The sound of the breath itself is considered a sacred mantra of power that is capable of revealing many secrets. Yogis have asserted a direct relationship between a person's breathing potency and his or her life force and personal power.

At the moment of birth the breath enters our lungs as we separate from our mothers, and the breath's final departure marks our death. Our breathing animates and empowers all of our actions and movements, and reflects our every state of mind and every emotion, yet very few of us observe and study this foundation of life. Hatha yogis have pointed out the importance and value of working with and developing the bioenergetic system. They have shown that the breath not only reflects our mental and emotional states but also can affect them. We unconsciously use breathing in many ways. When we concentrate, we breathe very slowly and quietly, or we stop breathing completely to focus. When we listen to children, or an emotionally charged friend, we are on some level monitoring the quality of their breathing for feedback and information on their mental-emotional state. When we are tense or angry, our breathing pattern changes. If we cut or bruise ourselves, we often clasp the injured place and breathe attentively, making an ujjayi-type sound, to relieve the pain. If a loved one is in pain, we instinctively place our hands on the area and breathe consciously to direct healing energy to the place in need. Sometimes after a stressful situation, we need to "just breathe" to recharge or balance ourselves. These are a few examples of our use of prana and energy.

Prana refers to both physical and nonphysical, even psychic, forms of energy. Although the existence of nonphysical energies cannot be conclusively proven, they seem to follow the same rules as physical energies. A mystic might say we are directing mysterious energy psychically when we practice, and a scientist might counter that it is faith or mental energy, but either way, something seems to be happening. Whether you believe in prana or not, pranayama works.

Breathing is both conscious and unconscious. The breath floats on the threshold of the conscious and the unconscious mind. We cannot even think of the breath without influencing it and without it coming back under conscious control. You can easily try this. If you're thinking of your breath now, you are controlling it. If you try to stop controlling it, you can't—it has to just happen by itself. Any attempt to stop controlling it is still control. I once had the opportunity to do some meditation research with a polygraph lie detector. While being trained to use it, I was shown that the most sensitive graph being monitored was the breath. Our slightest emotional tension is immediately reflected in our breath. Yogis discovered that our mental-emotional state and breathing both reflect and affect each other. We can change mental, emotional, and energetic states with the breath. This is the basis of pranayama.

All asana practice actually involves pranayama practice—whether breath work is done consciously or unconsciously. When the breath is left alone, the asana affects and creates the breathing pattern. It is best to learn about the effects of breathing in poses by experimenting and paying closer attention. Watch the difference in your postures when breathing softly or strongly, actively or passively, when breathing freely, or when using ujjayi breath.

One of the best ways to access the power of breath is with a pranayama practice. I have found that if students will take enough time, usually a few months of regular practice, to develop mastery of the techniques, and to discover their connection with their breath, the benefits can be lifelong. Once you have accessed your pranic, bioenergetic system, it will always be available to you. There are hundreds of pranayama techniques. The most important are *ujjayi*, *kapalabhati*, *bhastrika*, *alternate bhastrika*, *anuloma viloma*, and *sitali*. It is possible to learn a lot on your own and with good books, but it is best to learn these practices, and pranayama in general, directly from a competent teacher.

There are five different levels or stages in pranayama practice.

- Learning subtle control and mastery of the lungs and respiratory system. From our first breath at birth, breathing is our constant companion. It is rare to receive any breath instruction, unless as a singer, martial artist, or musician. Control and mastery implies learning to breathe both correctly and incorrectly, getting control over the diaphragm, being able to fill the lungs completely from the bottom up or from the top down, being able to fill the lungs laterally and even individually, and being able to inhale and exhale very slowly, and very evenly.

- Strengthening and recharging. The second stage involves learning to increase your breathing capacity and the strength of the respiratory system. The breath can be used to balance and recharge the psychophysical system. Yogis point out that the lungs are the inner sanctum of our bodies. There is but a thin membrane separating our bloodstream from the outside air, so it's a foundational principle of health and wellness to keep our lungs toned and strong.

- Changing the mental-emotional state. Pranayama can be used to relax, release tension, build energy, release fear or anxiety, and charge emotional batteries.

- Healing. We can learn to direct healing energy within ourselves and to others.

- Altered states. Advanced breathing practices can lead to altered, mystical, and visionary states of consciousness. Like any powerful tool, advanced practices require care, attention, and proper guidance.

In the early days of yoga in America, it was hard to interest people in asana practice. Jogging and other fitness regimes seemed more engaging. But, as people discovered, yoga practice can have far more depth and can be much more interesting and engaging than other fitness regimes. Working with the breath is similar. At first, it can seem boring or passive, but it actually has great depth. Many yogi elders have told me that over the years they found breath work as important, and even more important, than the practice of postures.

The breath is an entire information feedback system that lives on the interface of the conscious and unconscious, of control and surrender, the physical and nonphysical, fullness and emptiness, birth and death. When you learn to listen to and watch your breath, it is like listening to the waves of the sea. Like hearing the sound of a coming train or waves breaking, you begin to understand the subtle differences in modulation, frequency, and tone. These sounds convey information about what the waves are doing, their strength, how the water is spreading across the sands, and the breakdown of the wave as it crashes on the shore. You can discover and sense the messages and teachings in the sounds and qualities of the breath—the life force ebbing and flowing within us. The breath can be one of our greatest teachers.

## Using Locks, or Bandhas

Several types of muscular contractions, called *bandhas* (pronounced buhn duh, and meaning to lock) are used in Hatha yoga, both in pranayama breathing and asana practice. The most important are: the root lock, or *Mula Bandha* (moo luh, meaning root); the chin lock, or

*Jalandhara Bandha* (juh luhn dah ruh, meaning water pipe); and the stomach lock, or *Uddiyana Bandha* (oo dee ah nuh, meaning upward).

Mula Bandha is done by contracting and holding the anal sphincter muscles while creating a lifting sensation that slightly firms the lower abdominals. It is important also to contract the pubococcygeus muscles at the same time. These so-called PC muscles are easy to identify and control because they are the muscle sets we use to stop the flow of urine. They normally contract in tandem with the anal sphincters. Simply contracting and firmly holding the root sphincters should call all the necessary muscles into play.

Some Hatha yoga lineages advise holding Mula Bandha during the practice of asanas, and of course there are varying opinions. I have experimented and found many benefits to holding this lock during many postures or movements. It strengthens the abdominal muscles, tones the sexual organs, increases heat and concentration, builds upward moving energy, and can protect the lower back. Mula Bandha can be applied during any posture and even used throughout an entire yoga session. I have often found, however, that even when students try to hold Mula Bandha continuously, they in fact are holding it intermittently. When you are trying to hold it, you will notice from time to time that you have let go. Simply begin holding the lock again. You can also practice contracting and releasing Mula Bandha with twenty or thirty repetitions a couple of times a day in order to tone important muscles and the sexual organs. I don't agree with those who say you must always hold the root lock during asana sessions. My good friend and mentor, Swami Venkates, had a great saying: "Always is always wrong, and never is never right." Rather than giving a series of rules and specifying asanas and times to use the lock, I suggest experimenting with bandhas, experiencing their effects, and determining when they are appropriate. With practice, patience, and attention you will learn the secrets of this lock in time.

Jalandhara Bandha is activated by pressing the chin into the jugular notch in the collarbone while rolling the tongue back to touch the soft palate. It is used in certain breathing practices, especially on retention, and occasionally in asana.

Uddiyana Bandha is a lifting or a firming and contracting of the abdominal muscles. It increases strength and energizes the postures. The lock is best learned from a qualified teacher because one can easily cause incorrect breathing if it is not properly applied. This is because when holding this bandha one may tend to stop using the diaphragm or to use it in a tight or backward-moving manner.

All three of these locks can be applied simultaneously during retention in pranayama to build strength, to increase heat, and to circulate energy flows. Uddiyana Bandha, augmented by Mula Bandha, strengthens the physical body, the musculature, and the energy body. This strengthening effect can be demonstrated with muscle testing, and a well known similar principle in martial arts is to hold the solar plexus area, called the *hara* point, firmly. Using bandhas during practice helps keep these muscles toned and activated so they function properly when needed by the body.

## Traction, Torque, and Leverage

One of the wonderful things about yoga practice is that it can be done almost anywhere. Many poses can be accomplished in only the space the body occupies. Yoga requires little or no equipment and the body itself becomes the player, the instrument, and the music. After you are able to hold an asana comfortably with good alignment, you can start experimenting with using traction, torque, and leverage. Leverage can be created against external supports, such as the floor or a wall, or generated from within internal alignments of muscle and bone. Using one part of your body to push on another part combines internal and external leverages.

Use leverage and traction to create internal torque and precise articulations of joints and muscles. These biomechanics build strength, create internal opening, and relieve compression. For example, in the Plank pose, Downward Dog, or Headstand, you can press against the floor to create more lift in the spine. You can also press your legs against each other to strengthen muscles and create an opening in the sacral area that releases back tension.

Becoming aware of and learning to use *isometric* and *isotonic* tensions is also very helpful. Isometric tension pushes against a fixed resistance so that the muscle's length remains the same. Pushing the palms together against each other creates isometric pressure. You can also use isometric pressures to learn how to press different inner energy planes into external objects like the floor or wall. For example, you can press an energy line up the inner side of your legs by pressing down through the arches of your feet to the floor. Similarly, you can create a line of energy up the outer edges of your leg by pressing the outer edges of your feet into the floor. To experience how this works, try holding a ledge, table, or sink with your hands, and then push, pull, or lean away to experiment with some isometric levers.

In isotonic movements, resistance remains constant while muscle length changes. Push-ups, chin-ups, and pull-ups are isotonic exercises—they use one's body weight as the resistance. Extend your arms out to the side and raise them slowly over your head while resisting with opposing muscles in the arms and side body—this is an isotonic movement flow. Graceful flowing movement often requires working with internally created resistance. Isotonic pressure generates different levels of intensity with your own internal muscular resistance. Work with and against your own muscular forces to build strength, intensity, and core stability.

When you begin using and experimenting with levers and internal forces, your body will communicate with you and guide you from within. Everyone has experienced this to some degree. When you feel tightness or blocked energy, you often instinctively start moving opposing muscles to gain leverage, responding to inner signals until the block or pinch is released. I'm sure you can remember a time when your neck or shoulders were tight or locked, and you instinctively tightened your neck and dropped your head and shoulders while creating an internal resistance to work against to create opening. Or you clasped your hands together and pushed and pulled to create a needed effect guided from within until you released the energy and tension. Learning to feel and manipulate internal nerves, joints, and musculoskeletal dynamic tensions and relationships is not something that can easily be taught, but realizing that this is possible will direct your attention and makes it more easily achieved. You are already doing this to some extent and you can expand and build upon this process in your yoga practice. You can become proficient at internal skeletal and nerve adjustment and self-healing.

You can also learn to use levers by experimenting with different pressures and resistances in postures. In different asanas try pressing, lifting, extending, tensing, and relaxing different body parts in different combinations. For example, come only halfway into your usual seated Forward Fold. Then try pressing the legs and back of the knees into the floor, using that press to help lift the chest. Grab your ankles with the hands and push with the feet while pulling with the hands to further open the spine. At the same time you can create more internal leverage and opening by dropping the chin and lifting the back of the head and neck. Taken together, all of these should feel good and create a lengthening and release of tightness along the spinal column. Try this right now, get the feel for this process, and connect with your internal guidance system. There are literally hundreds of ways to use levers and internal resistances. As you progress, learning to manipulate your muscles and joints with internal leverages and torques is essential to gaining deeper levels of efficacy in yoga practice. Once again, your own body will teach you many ways to use these internal dynamics when you simply begin to watch and experiment.

## The Nature of Balance

There is an ancient, often quoted, definition of yoga: *Samatvam yoga uchyate,* or "Yoga is balance." Many students of yoga seek to find physical, mental, and spiritual harmony and balance in their lives. But it is important to see that balance is not a static place to reach; it is a constantly moving equilibrium of relationships. This insight not only applies to asana practice but to all areas of life. Our own personal balance will not be found in systematized or formulated modes of living and being, but in developing a sensitive awareness that responds and adjusts to the shifting moment. We can learn and experience the dynamic nature of balance in any balancing posture. Try a pose such as the Tree, in which you balance on one foot. No matter how still and statue-like you become, you will notice that you are continually adjusting and reacting in the moment. We must sensitively listen, feel, and respond. Harmony, in the same way, implies attuning, listening within and without, mutual interaction, and working in concert with oneself and others.

Instead of seeking to attain balance, we are better directed to learn the art of balancing. Balancing involves correcting errors and then in turn correcting any overcorrection of error. When you start moving or falling too far in one direction, in asana or in life, exert a bit to the other pole. Refining this ability, you become more stable, and the movements and adjustments become more subtle. To an external observer you may appear to be still or "in balance," but from the inside you see there is continual adjustment within this stability. This is another form of movement in stillness and stillness in movement. Maintaining balance and equilibrium is one of the precious goals in yoga. Our busy, modern lives cause many of us to seek to reestablish wholeness through exercise, right eating, and inner work. It is all too easy to overfill our days with constant input and activity—all too rarely taking the time to find balance present in the world around us. Both ancient and modern wisdom point out that nature is a dynamic state of balance. Where can we better learn about balance and harmony than from close communion and connection with nature? Sometimes it takes going into the balance of nature to find the nature of balance.

## Advancing in Yoga

The insights and principles outlined here are offered to assist you in refining your ability to see and listen inwardly and outwardly, on deeper and subtler levels, as you progress in your yogic journey. This awareness is more important than merely attaining more and more exotic postures. Think of your yoga practice as learning, gathering, and developing the tools for a lifetime practice of self-therapy, self-healing, and keeping your body in balance—remembering that balance is not a fixed place at which you arrive, but a constant adjustment process to the circumstances of each moment.

Advancing in yoga is more related to refining than to attaining. If you want to know if you are advancing in yoga, ask yourself these questions: Am I gaining greater understanding of my body? Am I learning how to heal myself? Am I learning subtler and different ways of using the poses and how each asana affects the body to produce different results? Am I gaining an understanding of the energy fields in the body and how these energies flow? Am I beginning to get some control of my own autonomic nervous system and some of the unconscious processes of the body? Am I less rigid in my beliefs and less fixed in particular systems and structures? Am I alive and awake in my practice, constantly questioning and willing to vacate my position—figuratively and actually? Am I questioning, not only of others but of myself? Is my mind becoming more open, compassionate, more peaceful? Growing in these perceptions and capacities provides the necessary ingredients for the evolutionary process of alchemical transformation into radiant health, high consciousness, and wisdom.

CHAPTER 6

# Useful Styles and Modes of Practice

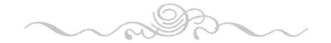

Yoga incorporates a marvelous body of knowledge, practices, and techniques. For any individual, some of these practices can be incredibly effective, others must be undertaken with great care, and still others should perhaps be cast aside. A particular asana or movement that benefits one person greatly may or may not be as suited for another. The task in practicing yoga is to learn various forms and modes of the practice and then apply them effectively and sensitively for ourselves in order to keep our psycho-physical-spiritual organism operating at the best levels for our particular body type, the activities we engage in, and the lifestyle we love. That relationship between the individual and lifestyle changes and evolves through the different cycles, phases, and stages of life, through the different seasons of the year, and even through the activities of each day. We need to relearn to dance life's dance with wholeness, wellness, clarity, insight, and love—growing our practice so that it adds more dimensions and levels of attunement, awareness, and understanding to life. One of the meanings of being *multidimensional* is learning to see and understand the appropriate uses of the many different dimensions of all things.

## Flow Yoga

Flow yoga, also called *Vinyasa Flow,* has become one of the most popular forms of Hatha practice in the world today, so it is important to examine some of the meanings and implications of flow. When we think of *flow,* the first thing that comes to mind is the flowing quality of water. Most people tend to think of flow in terms of adjusting and being pliable and flexible with circumstances and to the moment, like water adjusting as it goes down a steep canyon. But less immediately obvious is the fact that water needs something to flow through or upon. You cannot have the flow of liquid without the firm, supportive structure through which it flows. The interaction between the hardness of structure and the fluidity of liquid creates flow. Inherent in flow, and the lessons we may glean from it, are also the lessons of using structure and form. The interplay of structure, rigidity, and form with formlessness make up the movement of life.

Flow yoga usually implies an asana practice in which the movements link fluidly together in a graceful manner with a meditative awareness and attention to breathing. Flow yoga can be practiced in a vigorous, dynamic, and stimulating manner and also as a soft, gentle, restorative practice. Flow is sometimes misinterpreted to mean keeping up continuous movement without holding poses. Constant movement may be used when needed and desired, but individual asanas may also be held for long periods of time in a flowing practice. The dynamic flow of breath and energy continues uninterrupted during the external stillness of the pose, much like peaceful but powerful eddies of the strong river. Flow yoga implies a practice with a theme or purpose with poses linked or associated together. Many possible themes can guide the practice—relaxation, recharging, strength building, endurance, structural alignment, various therapies, focusing on specific bodily areas, enjoyment, or a complete practice, to name a few. Flow yoga uses proper body alignment, attunement with breath, focused attention, and development of a balance of strength, flexibility, and endurance.

Being in the flow also informs us to stay fresh and alive, like a river, and to stay in touch and present with the flowing changes of the moment in our practice and in our life. The meaning of Flow yoga also implies learning to practice and to "get into the flow" with what is appropriate for our own body in the moment. Most of us live inactive and overly sedentary lives, and we don't move many of our muscle sets and joints. A good, well-balanced yoga practice will stretch every muscle, move every joint, and work all ten psychophysical systems in the body to build strength, flexibility, endurance, firmness, softness, upward moving energy, and downward moving energy, while bringing a balance between the feminine and masculine within each of us.

The *Flow Series* yoga practice contains all seven classes of asana discussed later in this chapter. This series is designed as a complete, core yoga practice that can be used regularly. It incorporates a full complement of postures that are accessible to most students and the sequence incorporates the most important asanas and their counterposes. It is designed to build strength, flexibility, and endurance quickly and to provide a well-balanced yoga practice.

We have already discussed creating a balance and interplay between what we called inner-directed practices and outer-directed practices. Outer-directed forms rely more heavily on established sequences and structures. Inner-directed practices are more intuitive and concentrate more directly on listening and responding to the needs and impulses of the body. Both types are useful and have their strengths and benefits. A well-balanced practice draws from inner- and outer-directed approaches. As we advance in yoga, we learn to use these modalities more appropriately to serve well-being and wholeness. We must also remember that part of the flow is the ebb. Off time, rest, and even periods of nonpractice can be an essential part of balance, long-term flow, and learning.

## Intuitive Flow Yoga

A powerful form of healing and balancing yoga practice is what I call *Intuitive Flow yoga*. Intuitive Flow is strongly guided and directed from within. In this form we try to get keenly in tune with the sensations and messages coming somatically from the body and let those feelings and the body's inner intelligence guide and direct our movements. It is easier to grasp this concept by seeing that we all have bodily experiences that happen naturally and that seem similar to this description. For example, when you yawn and stretch, usually your movements are directed by inner feelings and impulses. Try it right now: Simply create a yawn and stretch with your arms and let the inner sensations guide how you tense, move, and stretch. It is not hard to let inner bodily feeling create and guide your movements. For another example, recall an occasion when you have had slightly cramped muscles or pinched nerves. When this happened, you probably spontaneously tensed, stretched, and moved, or even contorted, in an unpredictable manner, guided from within, until you felt what was needed to get back into alignment. These are examples of Intuitive Flow. In this yoga form, you create and emphasize these qualities until they guide your practice.

Intuitive Flow is more *feeling* guided than it is *thinking* guided—it does not use a lot of logic. For example, the poses and movements may not follow the usual principles of alignment and may not necessarily be balanced on each side. When you truly follow the body's inner guidance system, you cannot really predict how the movements will flow. They may not repeat on the other side of the body or they may be completely different by the time the flow gets to that side. That means that you cannot really do this form incorrectly. You create and move with the flow that the body's inner guidance system gives to your practice. The common design principle that form follows function can be useful here. The form of the posture is secondary to the functionality you want to create with the asana. Your focus is on the feelings and effects of the pose instead of the form and alignment of the pose. This form of practice has led to the discovery or birth of many poses.

To practice Intuitive Flow, start with inner quiet, emptiness, and inner attunement. Then let the needs and messages of the body unfold your practice. Usually this form is done slowly, with closed eyes, but even here, let the flow decide. You can get the process going by moving slowly, feeling any tight areas, and then letting the yawn- or stretch-like feeling arise and then guide the movements. Develop what I call a *healing feeling*, then focus on it, and follow where it leads. With practice, your ability to accomplish this will improve, and the practice will get better and more effective as you refine the process. Intermediate students who have a good feel for the asanas and who are in touch with inner energy flows will have the best results with this yoga form. It comes quite naturally. I use this form regularly and have taught it to many students who quickly find great value and wonderful results in healing, balance, and well-being.

One morning after an Intuitive Flow session, I took some notes that can be used as an example to understand the technique and help develop this type of practice. Here is what one morning flow was like for me: I started sitting cross-legged on the floor and noticed tightness in my back and shoulders. I clasped my hands and stretched them overhead. After holding the extension for awhile, energy began to flow through my arms and shoulders, but my back was still tight. I slowly leaned and curved my body to the left, held it, and then leaned to the right. Then I began to feel my body beginning to round and twist to one side and my arms followed until I was sitting in a somewhat rounded twist that released all the tension in my back. In a normal practice or class I would correct the alignment of this pose, but in this moment it was the perfect movement to get a release. Holding the position for awhile, I began to tune into some of the subtleties of the twist and the internal levers I was using. I pressed my knee into the ground, rounded my spine into the twist to increase the leverage along with the feeling of well-being and tension release. I continued to experiment with adjusting the pose to increase the energy flow and feeling of release, and ultimately discovered a new variation of the sitting twist in the process. After twisting, my legs seemed to want to extend into a long forward bend. I went into a Forward Fold and held it dynamically, but soon realized the "long" part of the urge was in my mind because my body seemed to want to move. I sat up and did a sitting twist with legs extended. This led to a Lunge pose and then into forward splits on one side. I ended up doing a sequence of movements on the left, followed by a similar but differing process on the right. So far I had been practicing about twenty minutes and I felt energized with a release of all the tensions I had started with. The process continued for another half hour and included some dynamic movements and long holding of certain positions.

Intuitive Flow incorporates and uses, but is also free from, tradition. If you are limited by a specific idea or definition of yoga, or a certain manner of practice and posture, creative discovery and new possibility are limited. Intuitive Flow is about listening your way into the practice instead of thinking your way in.

## Structural Integrity and Structural Archetypes

Developing an understanding of the concept of *structural integrity* will help guide your practice and your Intuitive Flow. In terms of yoga practice, structural integrity implies a movement or posture of the body that has strengthening, healing, and balancing effects and does not exceed the body's limits of stress or torque.

As you learn to read the subtle signals from muscles, joints, ligaments, and nerves, you become more conversant with the information systems in your body. Learning to use these inner information systems is part of becoming guided from within in your movements. It will give feedback and warning signals, so you will usually know before overexerting, overstretching, or overtorquing. I used the word *usually* to point out that no system is 100 percent reliable.

As our art and science of asana practice grow, develop, and are refined, the practice moves from an imitation of the classical poses from the past, or learned from others, into the fresh movement of discovery of *structural archetypes* in our body. A structural archetype is a naturally occurring, beneficial movement or position in the architecture of the body. These movements and positions are dynamically therapeutic and beneficial when properly executed.

Attunement to structural integrity and structural archetypes has probably been the genesis of most asanas in practice today. You can discover these movements in your own practice by attuning and listening within. You can grow and refine your ability to feel and follow the energies of healing and well-being in your own body. Then begin to adjust your poses by tuning in to the structural integrity of the posture or movement you are using. When experimenting with this integrity of action in your body, you will naturally come upon many beneficial asanas and movements. Generally, it is better to first learn what structural integrity and balance feel like in the body from proper instruction and practice before experimenting and improvising.

## Active and Passive Holding

Dynamic holding of asanas is an important mode of practice. This mode can be used in most postures and provides many unique benefits in a short period of time; thus, it is an important mode of practice in which to become proficient. Dynamic holding implies executing the asana actively in a way that, simultaneously and harmoniously, activates and sends energy through as many nerve circuits and muscle sets as possible while keeping attention expansive, all-inclusive, and in touch with all of these areas. Practiced in this manner, even simple poses like the Tree or Standing Forward Fold can become extraordinarily useful and effective. A simple pose can become more healing, energizing, toning, and enlivening while bringing many other benefits to the psychophysical organism. For example, *Paschimottanasana,* the Seated Forward Fold (sitting on the floor, legs extended, and folding forward over your legs), can be done passively or actively. To hold this pose actively, depending on your abilities, you might extend energy through the legs, pull the toes back, press the backs of the knees to the floor, lift the chest, drop the shoulders, extend the neck, and try to activate as many muscle sets as possible while holding the pose.

Passive holding, on the other hand, uses the minimum amount of energy and intention necessary to maintain an effective position or variation of a posture.[3] Passive holding implies allowing the body's natural internal spring tensions, circulatory energies, and kinesiological structures of the asana, to create the effects of the pose. For example, in the Seated Forward Fold, you would sit and bend forward, folding your torso in half at the hips. In a passive variation you might relax your legs, possibly letting the knees bend while letting gravity and the structure of the pose do the work and give the benefits. Holding postures passively gives unique, beneficial effects, and results not obtainable with other manners of practice. Even the Shoulderstand and Headstand have dynamic and passive variations with differing effects.

Rather than simply being opposite ways of holding poses, active and passive holding can be applied in a range of possible combinations at different levels. You can hold some muscle sets in a given pose actively while holding others passively. In our example of the Seated Forward Fold, you could dynamically work your arms and legs, pressing the knees down and lifting your chest while relaxing your lumbar in order to create space between the lumbar vertebrae.

You can learn to use passive relaxation and dynamic tensions of muscles and joints in different ways for different effects. Different amounts of energy can be moved through the muscles to get different openings and effects. Learning to listen in the postures, while experimenting with different combinations of activity and passivity, will greatly expand your ability to tune poses to desired needs and effects. It is better to learn to use this insight in your own body rather than to be given specific applications in certain postures. There is no one way to hold a pose and many shades of grey exist between active and passive.

## Long Holding

Some beneficial effects in poses are only obtained by holding a posture for a long period of time. The amount of time that defines a long hold is relative and subjective, depending on the difficulty of the posture and the ability of the practitioner. A long hold can be from thirty seconds or a minute to several minutes. Holding asanas for longer periods of time can allow deeper openings, releases of deeply held stress or tension, and release of holding patterns in the musculature that lead to better alignment of muscles, bones, and nerves.

Long holding allows you to penetrate into deeper and subtler areas of the body, to tune into more subtle levels of the dynamic of the pose, and to learn to use torque, leverage, energy flows, and openings that occur. How long to hold is directed by tuning into the effect and the release you are receiving as well as to the qualities of energy and other messages from the body that will guide the movements needed to strengthen, heal, or balance a given structure or complex of structures. If you only practice with constant movement and short holding, you cannot take advantage of the unique benefits of long holds. Many principles in other chapters and particularly in the chapter on pain and injury offer guidance in the application of long holding.

## Odd-Day Practice

Most people have a favored side in sports or habitual movements; that side is stronger, more flexible, and more focused. It is easy to develop the habit of practicing on the better side first and holding poses on that side for longer periods. This is because we gravitate toward the things we excel at. A good trick to counterbalance this tendency is to practice on the weaker or tighter side first.

You might find, for instance, that a forward bending, twisting, or balancing pose is much better on your right side than on your left. If you do your strong side first, you have an unconscious tendency to try forcing the weak side to the same level and may overly push yourself. You might get frustrated when doing your weak or tight side after the strong, flexible side and tend to spend less time with it. If you do the weaker side first, however, it is easier to devote more energy to it. Moreover, if you do the weak side first, you can always do it again after doing the strong side, to give the weak side extra attention to help bring it into balance sooner. A tool many yogis have found useful is to focus on their difficult side, their *odd* side, on odd-numbered days of the week.

## Car Yoga

A wonderful attribute of yoga is that many elements of the practice can be applied in many unexpected places. Friends may think us foolish or fanatical when we do yoga poses in a car, but some postures can be very beneficial, especially on long drives. In the early seventies I toured the USA to give yoga lectures and demonstrations. A friend and I drove thousands of miles in a station wagon and I adapted a fairly complete practice that could be done in the back of the car while he drove. I am sure many other yogis have done similar things. I also created some movements to use while driving myself that keep my spine from cramping and tightening.

You can do the same. One of the most useful movements while driving is a snaking practice. Use your grip on the steering wheel along with a gentle press of the heels for support and snake your spine around by rocking your pelvis forward and backward, side to side, and in clockwise and counterclockwise circles. As you do this, let these motions translate up and down the entire spine. A few minutes of this practice lubricates and hydrates the spinal disks and releases compression and tension. Similarly, twist your pelvis from side to side a few times and then roll your shoulders in circles. These movements can transform a road trip from a body-stressing event of spinal compression, to a body-balancing yoga session. Obviously you must be careful and attentive and should not do anything that compromises your driving abilities.

## The Neck and Lumbar

The neck, or cervical spine, is one of the most mobile areas of the body. We constantly turn and move our heads around, and hence the neck is one of the first areas to show wrinkling and signs of aging. Since all nerves from the brain to the lower body pass through the neck, it has been referred to as the "Grand Central Station" of nerve trunks. This complex circuitry and intense flow of information and energy through the neck make it one of the body's major areas for tension and pain— hence the expression "pain in the neck." We have been animals for far longer than we have been *Homo sapiens* and we have a deep, primal drive to protect our necks—the area most vulnerable to attack by predators. When we are fearful, we instinctively drop the head toward the collarbone, protecting the neck with the jaw. We also round our torso forward to protect our internal organs. People who are emotionally fearful or protective often have the effects of this demeanor internalized in the body, with a rounded, hunched posture and a closed chest area. You can try an experiment now by stooping your posture, sinking your chest in, and dropping your head a bit. Sit or stand that way a few moments and notice the effects it has on your mental and emotional state. Now do the opposite. Sit tall, lift and open your chest, and hold your head high. Feel the difference? For another experiment, tighten your neck a little bit, slightly tense your jaw, and just hold that awhile. Feel the tension's effect on your mind and emotions, almost like a state of anger. We all have some amounts of stored tension in the body. If it is chronic we probably will not feel it until it is released with yoga or body work. Doing the Shoulderstand helps free the cervical spine and release neck tension; backbends help open the chest, improve posture, and strengthen the mental-emotional body.

During yoga practice you can learn to break the habit of holding tension in the neck area. By paying attention to the cervical spine during various poses, you will notice when you unnecessarily tense the neck; then you can break that pattern. When learning to let energy flow through the cervical spine and develop neck freedom and awareness during asana practice, you will naturally carry the experience over into your day.

The cervical and lumbar spine areas tend to reflect and affect each other. Tension in the lumbar can translate up the spine into the neck, and vice versa. The lumbar is another major nerve trunk area and it has the additional burdens of supporting the torso, absorbing the shocks of movement, and supporting any loads we carry. Proper movement in forward bends, backbends, and twists is the key to keeping the lumbar healthy, as is developing an understanding of the dynamics of this area and the relationship of the hamstrings, psoas, and quadriceps.

## The Psoas, Quadriceps, and Hamstrings

The psoas, quadriceps, and hamstrings are key muscle groups and it is very important to learn about their relationship to spinal health and balance. When these muscles are overly tightened, they can cause back pain and immobility. The effects these muscles have on the pelvis also reflect up the spine into the thoracic and the cervical areas.

Most people are not even aware of the existence of their psoas muscles because they are rarely discussed and are not visible or tangible where they reside inside the torso and pelvis. The psoas are two very strong muscles that attach to the side and toward the front of the twelfth thoracic vertebra and all of the lumbar vertebra. From there they travel down through the pelvis to attach to the top of the femur, or thighbone. Because the psoas lift the legs, flex the spine, and rotate the hips, they are involved in nearly every asana. Many of us, especially athletic and active people, have very tight and shortened psoas and hamstrings, because these muscles are constantly used to walk, run, dance, and lift. Tight psoas muscles can pull on and cause pressure in the lower spine. The hamstrings connect from the back of the knee to the sit bones. The quadriceps are the large four-part extensor muscles at the front, or top, of the thighs. The quads work in concert with the hamstrings and psoas to move the legs and mobilize the hips.

When you bend forward, the limiting factor is usually inflexible hamstrings. If you sit or stand and start folding in half from the hips, you are only able to keep your back straight as long as the hamstrings have the flexibility to lengthen. As soon as the hamstrings are taut, you can only continue forward by bending and rounding the spine. If you pull downward and forward too aggressively, the give will usually have to come from the posterior spinal joints, which can undesirably weaken ligaments. This is why it is important to slowly stretch out and lengthen the hamstrings over a period of time. People who have overly shortened hamstrings are likely to stress the posterior spine every time they bend forward or pick something up. This is one of the common causes or aggravators of low back pain. Loosening the hamstrings is part of the formula for relieving back pain, as long as the forward bends are done without aggravating the posterior spine. Flexible hamstrings are crucial to mobility; hence the expression "hamstrung" is used to denote hindered efficiency and frustration.

Similar to the way hamstrings limit forward flexion, when you bend backward the limiting factors are usually tight quadriceps and psoas. When you start bending backward, the ability to tuck the tailbone, rotate the pelvis back, lift the chest, and take the foundation of the back extension down into the hips and legs will be limited by tight or shortened quads and psoas. These muscles must lengthen to allow the pelvis, chest, and spine to lift and extend backward. Stretching and lengthening these muscle groups can have amazing, beneficial effects on hip and spinal mobility and help relieve and prevent low back pain. I've seen this time and again with students and have experienced great benefit myself through keeping these muscles long and flexible by stretching them on a regular basis. Poses like the Lunge, Reclining Warrior, Upward Dog, and even simple backbends can be used to bring flexibility to these muscle groups. You may have enough information here to learn properly to work with and balance these muscle groups yourself, but if you are not clear about it, please consult a knowledgeable instructor.

## Seven Classes of Asana

At least seven types of asanas can be delineated. A complete and balanced practice will contain some form of all seven. These types can overlap each other, and many asanas contain elements of more than one type. Increasing your awareness of the different types and key principles of each type will help you to envision and design your personal practice.

### Moving Sequences

A philosopher once said, "Mobility is nobility." All life is movement and in movement there is great joy. While one of yoga's unique principles involves coming into a specific posture, and holding it without movement to get specific benefits and effects, Hatha yoga also contains moving sequences. The most well known are the various Sun Salutations. Many other moving sequences are made possible by linking different poses in Headstand and Shoulderstand cycles and in various standing series. Moving sequences give the most opportunity for cardiovascular work and they can teach us to flow gracefully and bring dance-like elements to our practice.

I first learned the joy of movement through swimming and experiencing the delight of gliding weightlessly through water. Later I found the same feeling in yoga, the pleasure of moving Sun Salutations, Headstand series, and Flow yoga. Many elder yogis have advised that to maintain our mobility throughout life, we must keep moving—"Use it or lose it." I've observed native peoples all over the world staying mobile into old age by keeping themselves moving no matter what the challenges. Movement is the basis of life and an important element to consider and to include in our practice.

## Standing Poses

Standing poses develop strength, grounding, and rootedness. They strengthen and tone the whole body, and over a period of time they prepare us for more difficult movements. Standing postures can provide a full range of movements and stretches that can give a complete workout. They can be practiced at the beginning, middle, or end of a session. They strengthen the nerves to the legs and teach the ability to keep attention over the entire body. They teach concentration and focus and bring awareness of the building blocks of geometry and bodily architecture.

In any asana, and especially in standing poses, it is good to build a good and properly aligned foundation from the base of the pose—from the ground up. Standing poses are good for warming up, building strength, learning symmetry and alignment, and discovering imbalances in the body.

## Balancing Poses

Balancing poses teach poise and equilibrium. The body finds balance through cues from the inner ear, visually, and from receptor sites located in the muscular and nervous systems. One of the great lessons balancing poses demonstrate is that balance is not a state or place to arrive at, but involves constant attunement, correction, and adjustment to changing conditions of the moment.

It is easier to maintain balance than to regain it once lost. When practicing balance poses, we need to move slowly into deeper levels of the posture. Don't proceed faster than your ability to maintain stability. Your stability will gauge how far and how fast to move into the pose—another lesson also applicable to life.

## Backbends

Backbends warrant special attention and explanation. They are, in a sense, the most *unnatural* positions for the body. By unnatural, I mean that we only rarely bend backward in our normal, daily movements. Our bodies are mostly oriented in various degrees of forward bending. Sitting, walking, lifting, running, biking, and the majority of our movements are essentially forward bends. The only backward stretch many people receive is if and when they lie on their stomachs propped up on elbows to read. For other primates, swinging through the trees gives a regular interplay of forward and backward movements that help maintain spinal balance. Living without back extensions is a major contributing factor in back pain, stooped shoulders, poor posture, and a host of other spinal problems.

After birth we slowly grow and mature from the rounded child's positions of creeping and crawling to the upright, erect postures of the adult human—the only animal that walks upright. In this sense, backbends have been called "evolutionary" and "farthest from the womb." As we age, without the benefits of yoga, we slowly round and hunch forward and lose our ability to maintain an upright posture. Backbends, in a complete yoga practice, can prevent and reverse this process. Because we are not accustomed to bending backward in our usual daily movements, backbends, especially the deeper variations, require special care and awareness to prevent injury. Backbends have powerful, anti-aging effects. They help counter the negative effects of gravity. They stimulate the endocrine system, keep the spine pliable and balanced, and maintain good flows of nerve energy through the spinal column.

Backbends require the most attention and awareness in asana practice, so I would like to present some key points for attention. When backbending, keep in mind the following important principles:

- Always be fully warmed up before going into deeper backbend poses.

- Stay attentive and tuned into what you are doing and feeling. Backbending can distract you by altering consciousness, and you also can't easily see what you are doing.

- It is very effective and helpful to stretch the quadriceps and psoas muscles before backbends.

- Maintain a strong, well-placed foundation with the legs—or with the arms in inverted backbends.

- Keep the feet and legs as parallel as possible.

- Tuck your tailbone to help prevent overextending the sacrum and lumbar joints.

- Many people find using Mula Bandha, or contracting and holding the anal sphincter firmly, protective of the spine and helpful in back extensions.

- Bend evenly along the spine. Keep the chest lifted, letting the upper body take more of the bend than the lumbar area.

- Keep a gentle to moderate energy flow, or lines of energy, into the legs.

- Slowly progress from simpler backbends to the deeper variations.

- Don't overextend the neck. Avoid the tendency to lead with the head and bend it as far back as possible.

- Inverted backbends, such as backbending from Headstand or Elbow Balance, can be easier on the spine. The same is true for supported backbends over a ball, bolster, or the arm of a couch and for backbends from the Lunge pose. They keep weight and compression out of the spine.

- Come out of the poses slowly and attentively.

- Always remember to rebalance the spine after backbends by easing into forward bends and twists. The body's spring tensions will reset to the normal balance of forward bends.

## Forward Bends

Forward bends relax and stretch the muscles, soothe the nervous system, and tend to lower blood pressure. They relieve muscle cramps or tightness accumulated throughout the day or in other poses and improve posture and body alignment. Forward bends may be practiced at almost any time during a session. Most often the limiting factor in forward bends is tight hamstring muscles. Spinal health and balance require flexible hamstrings. The relationship of these muscles and the spine is described below. Leg muscles are built up and tightened by nearly all physical activity such as walking, hiking, dancing, and biking. It is important to include enough forward bends in your practice to counteract tightness in the legs and back and to regain and maintain flexibility.

Give yourself a long period of time to lengthen the hamstring muscles if they are very tight. Think in terms of many months, or even a year or two, to lengthen these muscles, depending on your age and relative tightness. Be careful to take the forward stretch in the muscles—not by overly pulling and flexing into the spinal joints. Make sure you do not pull your shoulders up toward your ears, shortening and tensing the neck. Holding the pose dynamically for a time and then relaxing more and holding it passively for awhile usually brings faster results. By including some simple forward bends, such as the Standing, Hanging Forward Fold, a few times during the day, you can accelerate regaining flexibility and get the benefits of these invaluable postures.

## Twists

Spinal twists relieve pressures on the spinal nerves, align the vertebrae, and lengthen the spine. They are used to balance the spine after backbends and after intense forward bending. Twisting poses can be done near the beginning of sessions, as well as toward the end of sessions, to release any residual tension or compression. It is important to keep the spine straight during twisting to ensure the correct effects. Rounding the spine while twisting can undesirably concentrate the effects of the twist into one or two vertebrae. It is usually best to lift the chest and sit straight or keep the spine straight during the pose. Twists can release and prevent nerve impingement and improve the flow of energy to the internal organs and legs. Twisting postures should feel good and bring sensations of releasing tension and pressure and a realignment of the spine.

## Inversions

Inverted postures such as Headstand, Shoulderstand, Handstand, and even Downward Dog are tonics for circulation. They tone the whole body, counter the effects of gravity, and balance the endocrine system. The Headstand, called the king of asanas, stimulates the pituitary and pineal glands and increases blood pressure. The Shoulderstand, called the queen of asanas, complements the Headstand and lowers blood pressure, balances the thyroid, and is considered the great tension-relieving posture. Inversions drain stagnant blood from the extremities, tone the internal organs, improve complexion and eyesight, and have many beneficial effects on the mental-emotional system.

If you cannot do the Headstand, the Shoulderstand will give most of the same benefits. If you are unable to do the Shoulderstand, you can get many of the benefits by placing your legs up the wall or even by holding the Downward Dog pose. Inversions can be practiced near the beginning of a session, in the middle, or at the end, to balance and restore energy.

# CHAPTER 7

# Injury, Pain, and Healing

Wellness, healing, relief from pain, and prevention of injury are primary motivations for many people to practice yoga. The long, lean muscles developed through asana practice are less prone to injury, use energy more efficiently, and heal faster. But even experienced yogis may overreach themselves attempting new poses, and it is not unusual for yoga students and teachers to become disheartened if they or others get injured from practice. In my early teaching days, I sometimes got discouraged when people would come to class feeling great and then pull something doing a pose. I would think, "Oh my god, maybe this person shouldn't be doing this yoga. Maybe he or she was better off before." Then I started observing more people and found that those who don't practice yoga had just as many, if not more, problems and injuries. They might hurt their back just by picking up a shopping bag, by sleeping in the wrong position, or by the way they carry their purse or child. Many things may cause the body to go out of balance, even to a point of injury. However, yoga practitioners who practice regularly and for a long period of time learn how to heal their own injuries and, more important, how to prevent them.

Our bodies always change, and go through many different cycles, strengthening, weakening and, as we have discussed, constantly changing internal muscular spring tensions in response to changes in our activity, inactivity, and lifestyle. Over time we can learn to develop and tune our yoga practices to create balance and wellness through the many phases of our multifaceted lifestyles.

Many people think they are not suited for yoga practice because they have stiffness, weakness, or particular physical problems. Back and joint problems run in my family. Though I was never naturally athletic, I was drawn to swimming and worked hard at conditioning myself. When I was about eleven, I started learning to swim in a large pool at the high school near our house. I loved it, so I went out for the swimming team when I reached high school. During tryouts, I barely made it across the pool and had to talk the coach into letting me on the team. I was always last and the older kids on the team would hold me under the water till I thought I would nearly drown. Somehow my tenacity paid off and by the time I graduated, I had won several medals in swimming. When I first started yoga, it was the mysticism, the philosophy, and spirituality that drew me. I had no idea about physical components of yoga, and when I heard about them, I was not only surprised, but thought it absurd that a workout could have anything to do with spirituality. I now feel quite fortunate that I encountered yogis who included physical practice in their definition of spiritual inquiry and growth.

When I started Hatha yoga, I was quite stiff, couldn't touch my toes, and already had some low back trouble. Many poses seemed excruciating and I struggled at them. Sometimes I pulled muscles or pinched nerves and I had to learn to work with and through those problems. My brother became interested in the physical aspects of yoga and started practice too, but every time he experienced some joint pain or ran into some difficulties he would get very discouraged, say he was not athletic, and want to quit. I tried to inspire him with my stories but he eventually gave up. His back pains, immobility, and body problems grew worse. Now I know that people will potentially have more injuries and more problems from *not* doing yoga than from doing it. No one wants pain or injury, but we should not let fear of it stop us from feeling the greater health yoga can bring.

It is not my intention here to prescribe specific therapeutic techniques for particular injuries. However, what I can offer may be even more useful and practical. I want to help you begin to shape a context and begin developing a process that will inform and guide you in working with any imbalance or injury. You can actually learn to receive your own body's feedback and guidance from any injury or physical problems. Specific recommendations someone else may make are only useful to a point, since every injury is different and responds differently, even when seemingly of the same type. For example, I cannot count the times I've been asked, "What poses should I do for low back pain?" Lumbar pain is one of the most common ailments we suffer. But even if ten people have similar problems from, say, degenerated or ruptured fifth lumbar disks, none of those degenerations will behave exactly the same, nor will they respond to prescribed poses in the same way. Certain general practices and treatments may aid healing lumbar problems, but what is most useful is to learn the process of listening to your own body's guidance system.

## Pain Is Your Friend

When we think of pain, most of us probably feel we would rather not have any. We spend a lot of time seeking pleasure and avoiding pain. Once I traveled in the Himalayas with a swami friend who headed an *ashram,* or yoga monastery. The swami was committed to service and operated a few leper ashrams in the nearby foothills, so he took me to visit a colony. His lifetime personal assistant was once an impoverished leper whom he helped to heal; later, together, they created this amazing service project. All over India I had seen lepers who were missing body parts and seemed to be wasting away. Leprosy is a horrifying and terrible disease that makes most people recoil or run away. I confess I was quite nervous about going to a leper colony, but it was a powerful experience (similar to the death meditation discussed in Chapter 9); I was moved and learned a lot. For our arrival the lepers put on a joyous dance in a dusty courtyard between their mud huts. There wasn't a lot of funding for their facilities and they slept on hard cots and wore torn rags. Many had dreadful scars and were missing limbs, fingers, or toes. I was shocked to notice that though they were all reduced to the same lot in life, they still segregated themselves according to caste and their former stations in life, much to the chagrin of their caretakers. The swami explained to me that much of the loss of body parts and the other horrors they suffered happened from loss of sensation and pain caused by the disease. The victims would not know when they injured themselves—they would not feel it—and therefore they suffered frequent infections and gangrene. Loss of pain actually makes us very vulnerable to further injury. Pain announces and guards the edges of our limits.

I saw something similar when visiting a methadone clinic with a therapist friend. She explained that many addicts mask or cut off their physical and emotional pain with strong depressant drugs like heroin. She also said many of the patients were very abusive to loved ones and further damaged precious relationships. Numbing their pain and damping down their physical-emotional feedback system led to self-destructive behavior. I began to realize that pain, within reasonable limits, was a friend we needed.

One time in Northern California, when I was about twenty-five, a friend and I were hiking in the rolling green foothills. We came into a beautiful glade and saw several horses grazing on the spring grasses. We were both experienced riders, but obviously not experienced enough, because we thought it would be a great idea to jump on one for a ride. When we slowly walked over toward the horses, several trotted away, but we were both able to hop on a lovely, golden mare. My friend sat in front trying to guide the horse by holding her neck and mane. The mare trotted around a bit, then all of a sudden noticed the other horses had moved far across the meadow to the other side of a ravine and she took off at a gallop. As we approached the ravine, we realized she was going to jump, and my friend panicked and jumped off. I was thrown and landed flat on my back. I could hardly move, but slowly made my way home. This was my first big injury and the beginning of a long process with my lumbar. I recovered in a couple weeks but my low back was more sensitive afterwards.

During my first year of yoga study, I practiced asana daily for ninety minutes, often morning and evening. I worked hard at it and within a year or two could achieve even the most intense backbends, twists, and forward bends. The Sivananda organization I was involved with and its head swami in America paid little or no attention to sequencing, structural dynamics, alignment, and physiological principles of kinesiology. The greatest emphasis of instruction was given to just achieving the postures, the more extreme the better. Attention was mostly paid to the metaphysical and spiritual side of the practice. I advanced quickly and often, after long periods of sitting for lectures on cold mornings and evenings without a chance to warm up, I was called on to show difficult backbends like the Full Bow, Full Wheel, or Handstand Scorpion to large groups. I was also taught the erroneous concept that it was necessary to lie down and rest for a couple minutes after performing each asana in order to "get the benefits." After barely warming up, this caused us to cool down repeatedly. We questioned the physical safety of this procedure and were told that we were doing mystical or metaphysical practice and therefore normal physiological principles didn't apply. Soon I began to develop back pain, pinched nerves, and other problems. I asked for guidance, but got no satisfactory answers, and was only told to rest a couple of days or to massage myself. The problems worsened. As I traveled around the country and to Europe giving demonstrations to groups and on television, my back would often lock up for days afterwards.

# There Is No Such Thing as Pain

One cold winter day, about 1975, as I practiced in my living room while feeling a bit cold and tight, a friend came in and asked if I would lift him up and give him a back adjustment. As I lifted him up into the adjusting movement, I heard a crunch and felt a pinch in my low spine. Slowly the pain increased and my back began tightening up. Not thinking clearly, I lay down, but as that cooled me off I tightened up more and the pain became excruciating. I foolishly went to the emergency room and was shot with muscle relaxants and prescribed painkillers and strong anti-inflammatory medications. For a month I had to stay in bed and could hardly walk. One day a teacher I had trained came to visit and said he had a great idea for my healing. I asked him what that was and he replied, "Why don't you try yoga!" I had to contemplate the irony of getting the insight I needed from my own student while I was lying in bed, and not using the knowledge I had passed on. I stopped the medicines and started one of my greatest learning experiences.

Initially, the pain limited me to only the simplest of poses and I could not bend much at all. Most curious to me was how some of my muscles did not seem to function at all, even though they had a range of motion. For example, in order to pick up something off the floor I had to use the wall or a chair for leverage and support in order to bend over. My body could bend over, within limits, but didn't have the strength or ability to do so on its own. I began to experiment as I moved up and down with the aid of the wall to see what was going on with the related nerves and began to understand subtle levels of my body's intelligence, pain, and feedback system.

I realized that there is no such thing as one kind of pain. I saw, instead, that pain is a language, an entire information system. When we resist pain, and lump it into one category we label "pain," we miss the many layers and nuances of information being conveyed. Pain is one of the voices of the body's intelligence. Pain is necessary and defines the limits and the edges of strain and injury. Some pain sensation messages demand us to "Stop!" while other messages tell us, "Yes, do more of that, but go slowly." In fact, pain encompasses a whole spectrum of physiological information that actually begins with our first stretching or moving sensations in the muscles and increases in intensity until we near our maximum range of motion, at which point the sensations become very intense and we call them painful.

You can experience this range of sensation and information in many movements. For example, take a moment and do a seated forward bend. Slowly start bending forward while paying careful attention to the sensations. At first these sensations may be quiet or subtle, but notice you receive information from them. As you move farther forward, you will feel more muscular resistance and probably what you could call a pleasant stretch. If you pay careful attention to this, you will notice it is actually a very similar feeling to a lower intensity of pain— that it feels like *a good pain*. Continue moving farther into the stretch and, as you near your maximum range of motion, the intensity increases rapidly until it actually becomes unpleasantly painful and even commands you to stop! You can try the same thing in most any movement, such as by simply and slowly rotating your head in one direction and listening to the sensations and feedback.

## Local Intelligence

As I watched and worked with my back injury, I noticed that every morning I awoke with pain and a lot of stiffness and could barely bend forward. Something in my muscles seemed to fight me and resisted any attempt I made to bend forward or to twist. I noticed that if I would move very slowly into a forward bend, holding it a long time, often for twenty or thirty minutes, these fighting, resisting muscles could be *coaxed* to relax and let go, and eventually I would be able to move fully into the pose. More important, by doing these long forward bends, the pain and tightness would be dramatically relieved.

I began to explain this to myself and actually experience it with a metaphysical, but fairly accurate, concept. The body organism has many levels and layers of consciousness. For example, there is our self-awareness and self-consciousness, the consciousness in the muscles and organs, the metabolic intelligence, and the consciousness in cells, nerves, and groups of muscles. I will keep this concept sufficiently simple for this example without debating or defining the ultimate nature of consciousness. I will call presence, thought, and awareness *self-consciousness*. Self-consciousness tells the body to act or move. To raise your arm, you merely think it and, voilá, the arm lifts. How it does that is mostly up to the *local* consciousness or intelligence in the muscles and nerves of the arm. If we had to know the muscle kinesiology and structural dynamics to do this, we would not get very far. Take a moment and extend your arm firmly out to your side—you are putting your self-consciousness strongly into your arm. Now remove this self-consciousness completely and let the arm drop and hang at your side as if it were dead. This experiment demonstrates how energy and awareness move into and out of different areas of the body. We take this ability for granted, but when we have injuries, it can be severely compromised.

Normally when we want to raise our arm, turn our head, or twist our torso, we simply think and the movement follows—the local intelligence carries it out. But when there is an injury, the local intelligence can literally seal off an area of the body and prevent movement, to protect itself from further injury. We might say "head turn right," or "torso turn right," and after a few inches, either from pain or actual inability to move, we cannot go farther. The local consciousness says, "Hey, I listened to you before and look what happened! Now, say what you want, I'm protecting myself. Push any more, and I'll yell really loudly." Injuries can create self-perpetuating feedback loops that exacerbate and aggravate the problem. For example, a person might have a slight nerve pinch in the neck from moving or sleeping incorrectly. The impinged nerve causes local tightness and tensing. Then, in turn, that tightening further irritates the nerve, causing more tightening. However, when we cooperate with the body's intelligence, moving slowly and sensitively, listening and responding to the feedback, the body guides us and lets us in, accelerating the healing process by bringing back circulation and mobility.

When I say there is no such thing as pain, I want to communicate the importance of not lumping all pain together into one homogenous entity that we resist. It is much more useful, and accurate, to see that pain is an entire spectrum of information and a language of the body, acting in a similar way to sound or music carrying entire spectrums of information. What we call pain really refers to a myriad of messages that can inform us and our practice as we learn to understand its communications. Sharp pains can mean "Stop!" Dull pain can mean to go slowly and breathe as we move energy into new areas. As I learned to listen and understand subtler levels of information from my injury, I began to see how these inner messages literally guided me to adjust my movement's subtlety and showed me the way to heal myself.

I remember the feelings and excitement of learning this inner process. In the morning I would awaken stiff and immobile from my back injury, and I would get moving with gentle forward bends and embryo positions. Then I would do a seated, Half Forward Fold, moving into it very slowly and holding the pose for ten or fifteen minutes on each side, surfing the edges of stiffness and flexibility. If I pushed too far into painful areas, my body would yell and cause me to slow down and recoil. This short-term feedback guided me and the intermediate-term feedback of feeling good afterwards confirmed the healing benefits of the movements I was using. Sometimes I experienced setbacks, which I realized were also part of the learning, healing cycle.

I recall having a great "ah ha!" and realization in spinal twists. I was still doing twists as instructed by my first Sivananda teacher—with a rounded back and not much internal, dynamic energy. This rounded form actually hurt and pinched my spine. But by listening within, I noticed that when I lifted my chest and spine as I twisted, and when I created internal leverages and torques by pressing and lifting with arms and feet, my pain not only subsided but was released. The body literally showed me how to recreate space in compressed lumbar vertebrae and relieve the nerve pressure and impingement. This inner process of listening to and working with the body's intelligence can be used and applied in every asana.

I began to experiment more on my own to help my back and improve my practice with sequences and alignments different from what my early teachers and swamis instructed. I learned to do forward bends and twists to release and balance after backbends and to keep the spine extended and open in many poses. The injury became one of my greatest asana teachers. I learned that, though my L5-S1 lumbar disk had degenerated completely, I could compensate by increasing the intervertebral space with internal leverages and torques and by strengthening the spinal muscle column. In 1976 I met and hosted B.K.S. Iyengar in Los Angeles, and his instruction confirmed and expanded greatly on my own discoveries about the internal dynamics of asana.

Doctors had told me to stop practicing yoga and said I would always have back trouble. Surgery was suggested. I continued with my practice and within a couple of years I regained nearly all of my flexibility and strength on my own. Ten years later I relearned the lessons of the body when I got too involved in the construction of our retreat center and re-injured my back by foolishly carrying lumber and ninety-pound bags of cement. This time, however, I was able to cycle through the injury in a few weeks instead of years by following the principles I had learned with the earlier injury.

I used to be hesitant to discuss these experiences with students. I was concerned that they would be disheartened with yoga and they might conclude that if teachers and advanced students received injuries, yoga must be flawed or detrimental. But I found that the reverse was true. Students were inspired to see how healing was possible, to realize that no one is beyond the possibility of error or injury, and to be reminded that we all are human. There is no magical technique or practice that will keep us free from harm, injury, or physical problems. Any of us may exceed our limits, push too hard. Holding on to the ideas that we are practicing magical or perfected techniques is what puts us to sleep. It is staying constantly alert and vigilant that will guide us in the right direction.

## Sympathetic Resonance

Healing and wellness also have components similar to tuning the strings of musical instruments. *Sympathetic resonance* is the phenomenon where one plucked string will also cause others strings in the area that are in tune to vibrate. When we are sick or injured, other old injuries and problems tend to resonate with the current one and get set off again. For example, if you hurt an ankle, an old neck injury may start bothering you. Fortunately, the converse is also true. When you have a problem or injury and do what feels good with a practice that gets your energy moving, you will set up a *healing resonance* that helps the injured areas come back into alignment and wellness. By creating a strong enough field of well-being and mental intention, you can bring the whole body into this beneficial resonance.

It is important to trust your inner senses and to learn to listen and respond. You must be very careful not to push too far into painful areas during early or acute stages of an injury—to stay in back of the edges of pain until you are more confident. Competent teachers can demonstrate these abilities to some extent, but they cannot actually teach them to you. You must learn them for yourself. It is not difficult, though; just begin by listening and tuning in.

Dealing with injury is not that different from the way you should approach your entire yoga practice. Listen and respond to guidance from the body's intelligence, assisted by the knowledge and information as well as the techniques and modalities you have learned, in order to create a process that accelerates healing of the body.

## Causes and Prevention of Injury

Injuries have many possible causes. Increasing awareness of these causes will aid in prevention. Here are several of the most common types of injury, and ways to avoid what causes them.

### Accidents

We are all subject to unexpected injury. Yoga practice not only helps prevent injuries, it also trains us to accelerate healing. The following story shows how yoga makes the body far less prone to injuries. Once, when learning to ski, I came down a beginner's slope next to the lift lines. Watching the people in line and not paying attention to my skiing, I caught the edges of my skis in a wide snowplow and my feet and legs went out sideways until they were in wide, standing straddle splits. It looked like I would split in half and the people in line gasped. But I was flexible, and had even done the straddle splits that morning, so I was able to readjust my legs, aim the skis together, and pull back into the proper position as I skied by the line of shocked-looking people at the lift. My body had just said, "Oh, we're doing these straddle splits again," and I avoided what could have been an unpleasant injury.

### Congenital Weaknesses

Our heredity can leave us with known or unknown physical weaknesses. Yoga practice aids in discovering and learning about these areas and also in strengthening and bringing them into balance. Similarly, old injuries and traumas may still be stored in the body and as you progress deeper into poses they may surface again in the process of healing and rebalancing the body.

## Aggressive Practice

No one wants to be left behind, and we all want to make good progress in our practice. Pushing through limitations can bring some benefits, but you must also have sensitivity and take care to learn your limits without letting enthusiasm get out of hand. Pushing through a challenge must be balanced by paying attention and knowing when to back off.

## Irregular Practice

Once you have established a good yoga practice over a long period of time, you will usually be able to quickly reestablish your normal abilities after missing some days or even months. Of course, consistent practice is better, but life often has other plans. Try to be as consistent as possible and work back slowly to your normal levels after a long hiatus. Injuries can also be caused by cooling off from starting and stopping practice within a given session. If you must stop for an important reason during a session, warm up and ease back in the flow. Practicing unconsciously and mechanically can lead to injury. It is important to stay warm, tuned in, and to practice with awareness, according to the body's own limits. Demonstrating poses to friends or students, without being warmed up, can also cause injury. Teachers must also be careful if they demonstrate incorrect ways of doing poses. Lifting and adjusting students into postures is another area where teachers must be careful not to strain their backs and joints.

## Old Injuries

A well-thought-out asana practice eventually works its way into every nook and cranny of the body. Where there are old injuries, adhesions, weaknesses, or scar tissue, the asanas will sometimes cause the injury to resurface as the body is healing and restructuring. Be careful to move very sensitively and gently when working with old injuries. It's also important to consult an experienced body therapist or yoga teacher and use the internal feedback system described in this chapter to work with injuries.

## Other Causes

We have already discussed many other important tenets of practice in the Ah Ha! chapter. Whatever the difficulty, weakness, or injury, your yoga practice can develop beyond mere fitness conditioning into your own powerful, self-healing system, but it's important to remember always to deal with your whole lifestyle when looking for causes of difficulties. I forgot this once when teaching a medical doctor who kept getting headaches after his yoga practice. I experimented with various adjustments and sequences a few times in class before remembering to ask questions about his lifestyle. When I did, he told me that he drank ten to fifteen cups of coffee each day! He said he would cut back before coming to class, and this detoxification manifested the cause of his problem. After reducing his coffee addiction and drinking more water, his headaches ceased. No amount of asana adjustments would have helped him.

## Working with Injuries

Muscles, tendons, ligaments, or nerves can experience strain or injury. Usually the time it takes to heal follows in the same order. Depending on the severity, of course, muscle injuries tend to heal faster than similar-scale injuries to ligaments or nerves. Medical and physical therapists once advised rest, support, and immobilization of injured areas until they healed. Contemporary wisdom and experience has shown that getting an area moving again, as soon as movement is not detrimental, accelerates healing and allows the area to heal better, stronger and without adhesions.

Many therapists suggest an acronym, called RICES, to guide treatment:

- R is for Rest—resting the injury during the acute phase before it is advisable to start movement.

- I is for Ice—icing injured tissue helps prevent swelling and speeds recovery.

- C is for Compression—wrapping an injury can help immobilize the area and reduce swelling.

- E is for Elevation—keeping the hurt area at or above heart level helps with circulation and prevents fluids from accumulating.

- S is for Support—supporting the injury with a sling or taking weight off a strained area such as legs, back, or ankles with a crutch or cane.

RICES can be useful to guide you in using or administering first aid during the initial moments and first few days after a strain or injury. If the problem is not resolved and healed, then professional help as well as using the other principles in this chapter may be necessary.

Hatha yoga tends to be preventive, focusing more on health and wholeness rather than sickness, but it also is used as a therapeutic practice. A great teacher and information system, pain is not something we voluntarily seek out; nonetheless, it often provides a key catalyst in major times of learning and growth—both physically and psychologically. If we look back on some of our greatest experiences of growth and learning, we will find they often involved some pain.

Don't let injuries stop you. Learn to activate and assist your body's powerful healing energies. When working with sickness or injury, pay attention to any feelings of wellness and wholeness and give your energy to building and increasing them. Balance internal process and awareness with external input and feedback from teachers, healers, and body workers. Experiment with a good repertoire of poses and practices. You will not always find the right approach logically, as it often reveals itself serendipitously. You might just stumble on the perfect movement or asana by trying something new, taking a class, or letting your body guide you. An injury is a moving target, so your approach must be a living approach that attunes and adjusts to the movement of the process. We do not reach health and wholeness as a permanent, fixed state of balance, but as an ability to adjust continuously and dance with the changing realities of each moment. This living process will grow and evolve as it guides you through all the stages and changes of life.

CHAPTER 8

# Chakras—The Play of
# Matter and Energy

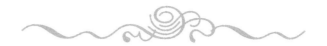

The chakra system (pronounced chuh kruh) is an ancient mapping of psychic phenomena and layers of consciousness. Though myth and folklore often date its origin back millennia, most academics believe the concept of the chakra system originated within the last several hundred years. Many view the chakras as having been "revealed," discovered or perceived intuitively, but scientific evidence suggests that their depiction probably grew out of religious practices and beliefs. Descriptions and definitions of the nature of the chakra system differ widely. The belief in this system may have started with external diagrams, sorcery, and the worship of goddesses, mystical beings, and power entities. The chakras have been described as wheels of energy, loci of power, and mystical power centers that exist in the subtle, or *astral,* body. They have been used as magical diagrams for sorcery or protection from demons, the appeasement of gods, and the control of supernatural forces or entities.

As it is viewed today, the chakra system has evolved through many, sometimes contradictory, phases of mapping and delineation often related to stages or levels of consciousness, awareness, and spiritual development. Various earlier chakra concepts have included four chakras, twelve, sixteen, and more. The story that this subtle, scientific "energy system" was discovered by mystics through inner vision is mostly legend. The currently accepted number of seven chakras was probably solidified in time and thought with the advent of the printing press and strengthened by the publication of Sir Arthur Avalon's books in England, *Kundalini* and *Sakti and Sakta*.[4] His diagrams and presentations of the seven-chakra system have become the most widely accepted. Avalon's seven-chakra system technically includes six chakras plus one, with the additional seventh chakra representing infinity and the synthesis of the other six. However, Avalon's chakra color rendition follows no apparent logic. Contemporary chakra renditions are often linked to the physical sciences, following the progression of colors in the rainbow from red to violet and pure white light.

Whether by coincidence, selective observation, synchronicity, or even divine revelation, the seven-chakra mapping seems to align holographically with many observable scientific principles. There are, for example, seven colors of the rainbow, seven days of the week, and seven notes of the musical scale before it repeats on the next octave. The seminal works by Professor David Gordon White, *The Alchemical Body* and *The Kiss of the Yogini*,[5] historically trace the development of the chakra system through the ages.

Philosophers and sages have debated about the origin of spirit and matter and the nature of consciousness for eons. Did consciousness arise out of matter? Did spirit or consciousness create matter? Or are they actually one and the same? The age of science has given much weight to the former argument—that consciousness evolved out of matter. The materialist viewpoint argues that the interaction of elements, energies, and sunlight created ultimately the chain of life from plants to what we call life's paragon—humankind, with its self-reflecting intelligence. Religious people have argued the opposite—that spirit brought matter into being. There seems to be no way to prove or disprove either position. The chakra model, however, shows consciousness and matter to belong to one interdependent continuum. Consciousness, or spirit, seems to require matter to express itself or to be known. Even an envisioned or perceived pure spirit realm contains a material component. To have shape, structure, space, and difference of any measure requires a defining structure. Which came first, matter or consciousness? It is possible that they are mutually embedded in each other. Matter, energy, spirit, and consciousness may be part of one interdependent interplay.

## The Chakras' Relation to Science

The system of chakras refers to a metaphysical or mystical aspect of yoga and Eastern philosophy. Being esoteric, the theory is difficult to prove or demonstrate and therefore easily lends itself to misinterpretation and misconception. Therefore, I would like to present an explanation of the chakras that is useful and practical (though less mystical) for the practice of yoga. After a number of years of study and experimentation with the esoteric aspects of this energy system, I began to see some direct correlations between the chakras, science, and various levels of experience and being. This proved to be congruent with mystical and spiritual levels as well. Early training in physics and science allowed me to find common ground between spiritual philosophy and scientific knowledge. I found correlations between the ancient chakra mapping, the energy-matter continuum, the periodic table of the elements, and the structure of the body.

The chakra system moves in ascending energy levels from earth, or solids, to cosmic energy. In a somewhat similar manner, the periodic table of elements charts how high energy coalesces down level by level from light, to gases, liquids and finally to matter. The chakra system can be seen as a holographic reflection of the cosmic continuum from matter to energy. It can also be used to map and explore the correlations of the movement from energy to matter with different levels of consciousness. *Holographic* has come to refer to phenomenon where the properties of a greater whole are contained or reflected in the parts. A *hologram* is a three-dimensional image made by the coherent light of lasers. Each part of the hologram, a holographic photo, contains information for the whole image. Fractals, geometric patterns that are repeated at ever smaller scales, are similar to holograms and are found in nature. For example, some ferns are generated by the plant repeating the same geometrical patterns, which build and combine to make the final plant structure. Each part contains the formula for the whole.

The word *chakra* means "wheel" and refers to certain *wheels* or *balls* of energy in the subtle or psychic body. Many ancient yogis believed that our physical bodies are animated by an energy body or astral body composed of subtle energies. This subtle or astral body is in turn created and animated by the field of consciousness. The chakras are seen as nonphysical energies that cannot be measured directly but that can be felt and experienced. To illustrate this concept, we might repeat the experiment from Chapter 7: Let your arm hang and swing freely from your torso over the edge of a chair or table, then withdraw your active consciousness from your arm and let it swing loosely like a pendulum. When the energy is withdrawn, the arm seems inert and almost dead. You can animate the arm again by directing your consciousness and energy back into it, even lifting it or swinging it forcibly. This is a simple way to feel how consciousness and the energy body is activated and withdrawn in your arm.

## Seven Energy Centers

The chakras are described as a series of seven energy centers located along the spinal column. The subtle body is said to be composed of 72,000 energy channels called *nadis*. In the same way that blood flows through veins, prana, or life force, flows through these nadis. They are similar to the concept of meridians in acupuncture and Chinese medicine. Of the 72,000, three are of prime importance: the *ida,* or moon, and the *pingala,* or sun, which balance heating and cooling qualities, and the *sushumna,* or "most gracious," which is the central channel along which the seven centers are strung.

At the bottom of our spinal column is the base chakra, which is said to be a coiled, mystical latent energy that can be awakened. This mysterious, latent energy residing at the base of the spine is called *Kundalini Shakti,* which means the "coiled energy," and is usually symbolized by a serpent. Serpents symbolize esoteric, hidden energy. Snakes live and hide underground and they invoke feelings of power and fear. In the East, *naga,* or serpent imagery, often represents esoteric, mystical, or divine powers. Many of the gods have serpents as canopied thrones, showing they have controlled or mastered these energies and powers. In the West, on the contrary, the serpent is often a symbol of evil, as in the story of Adam and Eve. The Western dragon actually better captures the ambiguity of the Indian naga than does the serpent. Some researchers have suggested that proponents of opposing religious viewpoints often recast the religious symbols of their adversaries, in this case the serpent, into symbols of evil. In any case, dragons, serpents, and snakes have always been powerful, evocative symbols.

The lowest and first chakra, called *Muladhara,* meaning root or base, is located in the sacrum ("sacred bone") and holds the latent, mystical serpent power, Kundalini. This first center represents the earth, or matter, center. The second chakra, called *Svadishhtana,* meaning "one's own place," is the water center. The third chakra is the fire center, and is called *Manipura,* which means "the jeweled city." The fourth chakra, the air center, is the heart chakra called *Anahata,* meaning "unstruck sound." The fifth is the sound center, called *Vishuddha,* meaning "the wheel of purity." The sixth is the third-eye center, called *Ajna,* meaning "the command center." The seventh and highest, is the crown center, *Sahasrara,* or "thousand-spoked wheel." One of the purposes of yoga is to bring awareness to these centers and to help awaken, balance, and keep them functioning properly.

The chakras are often described in great detail with specific colors, shapes, and numbers of lotus petals and associated sounds. Mystics have reported metaphysically seeing these wheels of energy in the astral body on the subtle planes. In visionary experiences we may see and experience the light body and many wonders, but we must use critical scrutiny to make sure we are not merely seeing our own inner projections. Energy manifests in myriad layers of reflective complexity. Psychological, physical, mental, or spiritual energy can also be projected through avenues of self-deception and exploitation. In other words, the mind can easily create and then envision self-serving, vivid manifestations of its own projections. Discerning the actual from the imagined or projected can be difficult or impossible and separating the two has been the subject of research and debate. In dreams and in meditation, we tend to see what we think about or elevate in importance. It is also possible to have true inner visionary experiences, seeing many layers of mathematical intricacy and geometrical relationship of matter, energy, and information as they integrate at higher levels of complexity and order. There are many ordered fields of energy around the body, and around and within atoms and molecules. Though the beauty of this holographic vision is ultimately beyond description, it nonetheless inspires many drawings of chakras, mandalas, and other artistic attempts at graphic representation.

"Awakening Kundalini" refers to awakening each person's seven latent spiritual and creative energies—physical/material, sexual/sensual, will/intent, love/compassion, expression/communication, mental/intellectual, and spiritual/universal. Awakening Kundalini can also be understood simply as awakening and manifesting our full creative potential. This understanding does not sound threatening, like awakening a mystic serpent in the spine, but it is essentially the same thing. As we have seen, power is neither good nor bad, but can be manifested or used in either direction. Releasing energy from the atom, or even by burning wood, is an example of the same kind of process—

freeing latent energies. Fire from wood can be used to cook our food or burn down our house. Used intelligently, it is quite safe. To awaken our potential fully, we must give attention to all the levels of consciousness being described in the chakra mapping. This essentially is the message of this map of the subtle body.

Understanding this subtle body mapping can aid in balancing our lives. There are people who "test" chakras and others who "read" chakras. This practice is sometimes possible and might be helpful, but we do not need to use a pendulum or a psychic to know ourselves. With self-observation and reflection, we can learn to discern whether we are grounded, whether we are balanced in our physical and material lives, if our sensual and sexual energies are off, if our love channels are closed and need attention, or if we have lost our spiritual connection. Some teachers speak of mechanical methods of opening chakras and their associated levels of consciousness. These methods may have some use, but are not complete in themselves. For example, to develop the throat chakra, the communication center, some people use certain postures, breathing exercises, sounds, or even crystals, but we must also learn to communicate and express ourselves in social contexts. Or, if sexual energies are blocked, certain postures, breathing techniques, and chants may be of some help and aid in focusing, but we will still have to work directly on the issues causing the problem. The chakras can be an outline, a metaphor, or perhaps a barometer guiding toward wholeness, but no map is ever the terrain, and we must always walk the actual ground of experience to reach insight and understanding.

## Chakras and Levels of Being

The chakras not only represent mysterious esoteric qualities, but actual levels of being in all aspects of life and in all areas of experience. The first chakra, the earth center, corresponds to the physical, material level of life. It is located in the sacrum, where we sit on the earth and where our bowels move earth out of our bodies. Being "grounded," keeping our "earthly" needs of food, clothing, shelter, and finances in order, relate to this center. No matter how high we get on the spiral of energy and awareness, we must always stay grounded back to the earth. We must have a connection or grounding and outlet for the higher levels of energy for which we become a conduit. Grounding implies keeping our lives in order on the earth plane within our bodies, our livelihood, and our relationships.

The second chakra, or water center, located a little farther up the spine in the area of the bladder, ovaries, or prostate, is the center of sensation, sensuality, and reproduction. Reproduction is an activity involving an exchange of fluids and swimming cells. Balancing this center involves harmonizing our sensual and sexual energies. The third center is the fire center of power, intention, will, and force. It is located at the center of gravity in the body near the level of the navel and corresponds to the digestive fire and solar plexus. This is the place where fire burns in the body, where our personal power resides.

These first three chakras, the lower centers, are considered centers of our basest powers. This is because if we function without being informed by higher qualities of love and awareness, we may be selfish, immature, or even violent. We may be motivated solely for power, sensation, or acquisition. The power center can dominate the sexual or earth levels. Working with this level involves balancing personal power. Power, we know, has an enormous potential to corrupt. The more power we have, the more self-examination and introspection we need to have integrity with the potential of that power. Similarly, the more power someone outside of ourselves has, the more scrupulous and watchful we must be in questioning and critiquing that person.

The fourth wheel of energy, the heart or air center, corresponds to the lungs and heart in the body. Opening this center implies the awakening of love and compassion. The heart and chest area are where we breathe and feel love, spirit, and compassion. This chakra is considered the first of the higher centers—with love, everything in life resonates at a higher level. At this center we transform from the lower level of the love of power, to the higher level of the power of love. This chakra is considered the source of music, even though the next, the fifth, is the center of sound. The heart chakra also represents the power of music to transform and open the heart.

Located in the throat area, the fifth chakra represents sound and communication across space. Clarity of speech and communication, writing, and poetry are qualities of this level of being. Sound carries unique qualities of feeling and information. A simple statement can communicate many levels and layers of information with differences in the tonal quality, pitch, volume, and modulation of sound. The sixth chakra is the center of consciousness. It is also called the third-eye center and corresponds to the frontal lobes of the brain and the mysterious pineal gland. This gland performs many known and unknown functions and can release hormones and neurochemicals during birth, death, and moments of intensity that unlock pathways in the brain, bringing mystical experience and transcendent perceptions. This chakra is the light center of awareness, thought, psychic power, and perception.

The seventh chakra, which corresponds to the crown of the head, is also called the thousand-petaled lotus, which symbolizes infinite energy. It represents cosmic consciousness and the union of all polarities and the godhead. Some say this center is the source of the expression "seventh heaven." This center is both a chakra and not a chakra: It is everything and nothing, unity and diversity, male and female, the union of god and goddess, the One. Seated in this chakra, the god Siva and the goddess Shakti exist in sexual union, representing both oneness and duality. This center connects us with all that is.

Substantial evidence supports the theory that the universe is holographic. This means that in some way each part contains a pattern of the whole. Chakra theory, it turns out, corresponds to the patterning and play of energy in the physical universe. One of the first things we learn in the study of electronics is that electrical energy is in fact a polarity, a potential difference. A battery, for example, must have a positive pole containing a deficiency of electrons and a negative pole containing an excess of electrons. The stored power of the battery is the polarity, or potential, of the excess wanting to return to the deficiency. Matter and energy may represent the ultimate polarity. At the center of our own galaxy, the Milky Way, we have an enormous concentration of energy, most readily experienced as light. As this energy moves out from the galactic center, it "cools" or condenses into lower levels of vibration, creating all forms of matter along the way. Some of the steps in this movement are expressed in the patterning of matter graphed in the periodic table of the elements. Each step across the periodic table represents the incorporation of greater levels of energy into the atomic structure. In a similar way, each step up the chakra system represents a higher level of energy.

## The Cosmic Polarity

Matter is essentially energy condensed to the point of having a nucleus with protons and electrons. Einstein showed that matter and energy belong to one spectrum—that they are in fact one. They are the opposite poles of a polarity. His famous formula $E = MC^2$ proved that there is tremendous energy stored in matter. The amount of energy is equal to the mass of the matter multiplied by the constant speed of light squared. This explanation has shown that the energy from the Milky Way galactic center is stored in the matter that makes our Earth. Triggering the release of this energy with the atomic bomb is a dramatic demonstration of this law. The bomb releases the many forms of energy—heat, sound, waves, radiation, and light—that was bound up in the form of matter and reveals the whole spectrum along the continuum between the matter and energy poles.

In Eastern philosophy, this cosmic polarity is represented by Siva and Shakti. Siva is the static masculine principle in the universe and Shakti is the active feminine principle. Shakti literally means energy. The dance between Siva and Shakti is said to create everything in the universe, which is, in fact, how all things are created by the interplay of matter and energy. The highest level of energy is considered the actual source of all things because it contains both Siva and Shakti, matter and energy, as well as the laws that allow it to become diversity. The mystic says everything is the mind of God. Many scientists say that at the core of atomic structure is information. Pure energy is both Siva and Shakti in union as one. When physicists designed experiments to determine whether light is a wave (a form of energy) or a particle (a form of matter), the result showed that, in effect, both are true. The answer is "it depends how you look at it." The way in which the experiment is designed and observed affects the outcome. (The philosopher, J. Krishnamurti, often stated, "The observer is the observed," as was also pointed out by the scientist, Werner Heisenberg, in his well-known Uncertainty Principle. The *Bhagavad Gita* talks about learning the difference and relationship between the "field" and the "knower of the field.") Light is both a wave and a particle, with qualities of energy or matter, depending how we observe it.

Regardless of how much energy or matter you remove from Earth, it remains essentially the same. This is because it is already one side of the polarity. When energy is added back into matter, it recapitulates the stages of matter's creation as it coalesced down from light and seems to follow the levels mapped by chakras. For example, if we slowly add energy to a solid, it remains essentially the same until a specific critical quantum point is reached; then it jumps to the next level or plateau—liquid. Continue adding energy and it goes through the stages of fire and gas. Releasing the energy of gas, like splitting the hydrogen gas atom, is the last material stage before a quantum leap that yields a release of wave energy (sound), information, and light that merge back with the oneness of energy. Earth-matter, water-liquid, fire-gas, sound-waves, and light are stages along the way. The seven corresponding levels, which relate to the chakras, are (1) earth-solid-matter; (2) liquid; (3) heat-fire; (4) gas; (5) dematerialization into wave energy or sound; (6) mind-thought, consciousness, information; and (7) infinity—oneness, pure energy, everything, and nothing.

Earth spins in an outer spiral arm of our galaxy. Seen in this way, the planet Earth is a cooled manifestation, or lower frequency, of the same energy that created it. Putting religious perspectives aside, we see that life is created from the interplay of cosmic energy and matter. This broad spectrum—light, cosmic rays, and energies irradiate the earth to create Gaia or the web of life. Microscopic plants are the first children of Gaia. Plants take the energy of the sun and combine it with the elements in earth to make life. In an actual sense, then, Gaia constitutes a polarized re-expression of light, which then creates its own self-reflecting children. The circle of light creates the circle of life.

## Chakras and Daily Life

Chakra theory holds wisdom applicable to daily life. Some teachers map the chakras like a ladder to climb, rung by rung. On the contrary, the view presented here shows how each chakra signifies an important level of being that operates simultaneously with all the others. We can work concurrently with all of these levels in ourselves. Electronic law teaches that for energy to flow properly it must have a ground. The root chakra's message is to keep your feet on the ground, to stay rooted and to keep your physical needs and affairs in order. The message from the water center teaches us to learn to flow and remain adaptable and to give conscious attention to sensual and sexual balance. Fire instructs in developing will and intention, and accepting change and transformation. Fire purifies and changes the form of that which passes through it. It is the doorway from the tangible to the intangible. The log in the campfire is transformed back into earth, sound, heat, and light. We must keep our personal power and fire stoked and alive, developing strength of intention and will.

The heart chakra serves as a fulcrum for all the other centers—the three higher and three lower. This center lies midway along the chakra system, where it can resonate equally above and below and balance the higher and lower. It instructs us to make the heart and love the center of our being. It implies that love should resonate through all the other levels. It is the balance of male and female. This center lies at the doorway to the higher planes and at the quantum threshold where matter transforms into energy. The symbol of this center, the six-pointed star made by the equal intersection of two equilateral triangles, $\triangle \bigtriangledown$ ✡ shows the meeting and balancing of the higher and lower, the masculine and the feminine. Earth rises $\triangle$ to meet heaven, and heaven descends $\bigtriangledown$ to meet earth through love at this fulcrum. Love is the turning point of materialism to spirituality.

The sound center instructs in communication and creative expression, as well as developing the ability to speak with truth, love, clarity, and poetry. The third-eye center inspires awakening inward perception, learning to look within. We have two eyes to look outwardly and a third that provides inner vision—"insight." The inner creates and reflects the outer. Inner vision leads to clarity of thought, intuition (to "see into it"), psychic energy, insight, and clairvoyance—"seeing clearly."

The highest center is above the Ajna, the command center. It is beyond our command or control. We exist by the grace of the Source. The idea of awakening or controlling this infinity is immature. We can, however, feel and perceive our cosmic connection with all that is. Silence is the quality of this level. Meditation, in which the observer dissolves and *is* the observed, is the realization of the thousand-petaled lotus of light.

The practices and concepts of chakra and Kundalini philosophy have been linked in origin to the long alchemical search for changing base metals to precious metals. Stills and other apparatus were used in attempts to heat, cook, and distill lead or mercury into gold or magical potions. This external process was eventually internalized to try to "cook" bodily fluids at the base of the spine and distill them upward through the spinal cord to the brain in order to gain magical powers or to attain physical immortality. The symbolic analog of this process may be far more important, however: Turning a leaden life into a golden life may be the real esoteric teaching of this form of yoga and the greatest of all alchemy.

CHAPTER 9

# Meditation Is Your Life

Your entire life is your meditation. All other specific forms of meditation technique are secondary. By integrating qualities of attention, awareness, caring, and insight into all arenas of living, we reach the deeper core and more essential meaning of meditation. This is an important contextual perspective to elucidate before proceeding farther in an inquiry into specific meditation techniques. Rather than simply asking how to meditate, it is better to explore first the essence of what meditation is.

## What Is Meditation?

Meditation practice is often described as the most essential and special aspect of yoga necessary to provide meaning and direction for ordinary life. We are often promised endless benefits from practicing meditation—from relief of tension and anxiety to much loftier goals including freedom, the ending of suffering, and enlightenment. But promising such lofty goals in describing meditation practices also gives them great weight and can make meditation one more source of pressure or conflict in our lives. We may worry about learning how to meditate and finding the right meditation technique among the myriad approaches. We can be troubled about whether we are meditating properly or for enough time, and whether we can control our minds. All these conscious and unconscious pressures can make meditation, which we have sought for peace, harmony, and wisdom, another burden we carry.

As soon as we ask *how* to meditate, we are thrown into the field of techniques and practices. Instead of limiting our discussion of meditation to descriptions of specific practices, I would like to point out two broad, general approaches to meditation. The first approach defines meditation in terms of specific practices, techniques, and more structured characterizations. This *prescriptive* approach tends to be mechanistic and arbitrary. Literally thousands of formal meditation practices—including repetition of mantra, prayers, or affirmations; gazing at candle flames, mandala drawings, or photographs of teachers or divinities; watching the breath, and many more—promise specific results. The majority of these formal practices can be characterized as *mind control systems*—learning and developing the ability to control your mind and thoughts, through the practice of a technique. Such meditation practices can be useful and beneficial, but the deeper meaning of meditation also implies a state of seeing and being and not merely a controlled *doing*—not another formal discipline. Our lives today have enough psychological difficulty and internal struggle and we certainly do not need to add more. How can we escape mental pressure through yet another form of effort and control?

Fortunately, meditation can also involve spontaneous awakenings of perception, artistry, and insight that inspire a very natural flow and state of being that pervades our entire life. It does not necessarily require years of practice, effort, and mind control. This second broad approach of meditation is more mysterious and indefinable; it sees the essence of meditation to lie beyond form and mechanical practice. This approach to meditation involves a living, evolving energy of perception that has a beginning, but no end, and no specific formal practice.

This "formless form" is without limitation and can take place any time, any place, and encompasses meditation as a quality of insight and awareness that, when awakened, can move through and integrate all parts of life. It is not desirable to give detailed description of formless meditation because to do so makes it into another technique. It is better to point toward this possibility and not give it too much definition. We begin to see all things in life as part of meditation. But this does not imply living in a controlled, stiff, self-conscious, nonspontaneous manner—it is quite the contrary. The formless can work through the form, but the structured can never become the formless. Understanding this broad dimension beyond form and technique is the most important foundation of vital and dynamic meditation—the meditation that is your life.

## Can Meditation Be Practiced?

If we were to ask ourselves why we wish to meditate, part of our answer would probably include gaining greater self-knowledge and understanding, growing as a person, growing in love and connection, moving toward wisdom and insight, discovering the mystical, moving into spiritual energy and awareness, and finding greater peace and harmony. I suggest that any and every activity in life holds the possibility of moving us in these directions and therefore all activities of daily life can be meditation. Everything in life has the potential of moving us to greater understanding and wisdom—and we cannot predict where the greatest lessons will lie. We may think of meditation primarily as sitting silently, but often our greatest growth and awakenings happen in the turbulence of daily life, in a moving experience, or in the magical colors of a sunset—and even in painful experiences. This realization is another way of pointing out that meditation can take place any time and is not limited to specific practices.

An old story may help illustrate this point. There was once a group of monks living in a remote monastery. Every few months they observed a very intensive sitting meditation practice wherein they would sit for sixteen hours a day for a week. One monk could not bear doing this yet again, so he placed himself at the end of the line as it filed into the dark meditation hall, and then slipped away as his brethren entered the hall. Going to the kitchen, he grabbed enough rice and apples for a week, then took his sleeping sack and hiked into the mountains until he found a beautiful meadow in a clearing. There he watched the flowers, birds, and animals, and each night he gazed into the cosmos. He contemplated his regimented life and practices and became absorbed in the beauty of the earth and stars. After the week, he felt completely reborn and renewed, and had a refreshing glow about him. He returned to the monastery just in time to rejoin the line of monks leaving the hall. As they all went to share a meal, the bretheren noticed the change and glow that had come over their fellow monk. They asked him to share how his meditation had been so evidently effective. What did he do? What technique did he use? He confessed leaving the hall and missing the intensive. After he described his experience in the meadow, the other monks leapt from the table, desperately asked him exactly how much rice and how many apples he took, and then they rushed off to find that meadow of enlightenment. Of course, they could not repeat his awakening.

When we look beyond static prescriptions and define meditation as anything that gives us self-knowledge, understanding, wisdom, artistry in living, awareness of the miracle of existence, and love, it becomes easier to see how this process can take place during any activity. Instead of meditation being one more thing to do and practice, everything we do in life becomes part of meditation.

Many define the goal of meditation as a silent, even empty, mind. But we must also realize that there are numerous other petals to the flowering of the mind, and of life, beyond the singular ability to have a calm or silent mind. The blossom in its fullness is made up of far more than one petal. While extraordinarily important, inner silence is still only one petal of the flowering mind. A vibrant mind, an active mind, a sharp mind, a clear mind, a penetrating mind, a questioning mind, an aware mind, an intelligent mind, an efficient mind, a mind that knows its own limits, a reality mobile mind, a flexible mind, a receptive mind, a free mind, a multidimensional mind, and of course, an open mind—these are just a few of the myriad valuable capacities of the mind. There is no end to the possibilities of a mind free to resonate at different levels and frequencies. Because our minds seem so overly active and agitated, the value of a silent, empty mind has been, perhaps, overemphasized. Considering other qualities and possibilities of mind reveals their importance and cultivates the ability to access different realities, and different states of consciousness. To have insight into your mental dynamics, structure, and inner nature is part of the essence of meditation, and part of life itself. The deepest insight will not come from studying someone else's sutras, though they may be of some help. Seeing comes into being through the study of yourself in daily life. Sitting meditation is only one part of self-realization. It is also important to develop a full repertoire of possibilities, levels, and dimensions of mind and not overly, nor exclusively, focus on emptiness and silence. Meditation is the exploration of the myriad possibilities of mind, all the petals of the lotus of consciousness.

We seem to be habituated to sanctifying instructions and prescriptions from the past. This is probably because prior to the modern era an ordered society depended on unquestioning obedience to elders and ancestors. Obedience to elders and authorities lies in deep strata of our social, cultural, and religious conditioning. Many modern yogis seem to have such a need for validation from past authorities; they feel it necessary to find justification, in past texts, for every discovery and every innovation in yoga. Patanjali's sutras, for example, are relied upon for answers to everything about life and therefore have been extrapolated in every possible way and stretched to include every possible meaning. These sutras may still hold useful teachings, but we must also acknowledge that these texts came out of archaic worldviews and do not have all the answers. For example, Patanjali had little or nothing to say about nature, relationship, and love, and he dealt mostly with areas of practice and mind control. The sutras, other ancient writings, and contemporary teachings can all stimulate and guide, but you must go through the doorway of your own self. Your own mind is the sutra, your own consciousness, your own life, is the meditation. Everything in life contributes to unfolding awareness.

## (There Is No) How to Meditate

It has been said that "meditation cannot be taught, but meditation can be learned." This implies that meditation involves subtle dynamics and not just mechanical practices of technique. Structured meditation practices can be useful and valuable. Sitting meditation can contribute with great value to inward awareness, stilling the mind, relieving tension; it can become a catalyst and impulse for creativity and new ideas. Sitting can be part of increasing self-knowledge and understanding, learning the nature of mind and thought, and entering the inner world. At the same time, it is wise to realize that any tool can be either beneficial or detrimental. It takes sensitive and careful awareness to perceive the appropriateness and usefulness of any practice at any given time.

Formal spiritual practices tend to be put forth as intrinsically good and always of positive value. However, we would be better served by understanding that all things can cut both ways, even if intended to have only positive effects. Spiritual practices, such as meditation, chanting, prayer, or even asana practice, can have beneficial *or* detrimental results. If we ask, "Is a knife good or bad?" The answer is yes—it is both. It always depends on the use and intent. There are certainly rules and principles about using a knife safely and correctly, but the real essence of using powerful tools is an indefinable sense of awareness and sensitivity in action in each moment. Although practices enable us to get better at what we practice, they can also lead to habitual, unexamined behavior or self-righteousness. Getting better at anything is also double-edged. Improved abilities can be used for good or for harm—there is no guarantee of always being one or the other. What is important, then, to one sincerely seeking spiritual growth is to keep attention on the feedback and results, both short-term and long-term, of all of practices. Once again, questioning and inquiry are a light to guide us along an ever-changing path.

We are better off, and more likely to use practices wisely, when we see that our mechanical techniques are not certain to lead us to greater awareness. If we look around, it is not hard to find people who have meditated for years and who have become more closed and more insensitive. Some who practice yoga and asana grow and blossom, while others harden and seem to regress. Realizing these differing possibilities is part of the light of awareness that increases the positive potential of the practices we choose to use. Developing our ability to question, to listen, and to be sensitive to the feedback and the effects of our practices is key. The vast unconscious, the unknown, the mystery of life, is not at our beck and call. We are not going to invite the infinite and control our destiny with tiny mantras, mechanical contrivances, or simple techniques of repetition. Repetitive practice and behavior quickly becomes automated and unconscious. Real meditation is more of a "happening," similar to sleep, or even love, rather than just something we do. There is no formula for falling asleep. Although you can prepare and relax, the more effort you apply, the less likely sleep will come. Similarly, while it may be important to prepare for love by being more caring, more sensitive, and less aggressive and self-centered, love comes when it will. Love is bigger than we are. A great teacher once said, "Every effort at meditation is the abject denial of it." We cannot *program* ourselves to love or to meditate. Meditation is more about deprogramming than programming. Meditation is not dull, mechanical, repetitive behavior chasing the magical, mystical, and spontaneous. Moving toward insight, wisdom, and clarity does not result from following systems, but from awakening. This awakened perception can act in all facets of life.

The majority of formal meditation practices involve self-control, mind control, or the perfecting of techniques and systems. Some define meditation as the perfection of concentration. Concentration, however, is only one power of mind and consciousness, and it comes naturally in direct proportion to our interest. We have excellent powers of concentration when we are very interested—just observe the motionless, rapt attention people exhibit for hours during good movies. Studying and understanding the nature of interest can be more useful than cultivating concentration techniques. Many people find the meditation practices that have been prescribed for them to be boring, and perhaps rightly so. If we were truly interested, we would find them engaging and absorbing.

Out of habit we look to systems and techniques for solution to problems. When faced with a problem or difficulty, we say, "What should I *do*?" Many areas of life, especially the technological and physical, involve learning and mastering techniques. But psychologically and spiritually we need space and freedom. When we live according to doctrines and dogmas, however sophisticated, we often sacrifice creativity and aliveness and become mechanical and automated. Real meditation must be a powerful solvent that penetrates the deeper layers of conditioning and programming to free the mind and consciousness to see farther and deeper than ever before. Meditation does not come from the repetition of the belief of another person or system. Awareness and personal understanding are necessary to neutralize and go beyond conditioning. To free the mind and consciousness, we must become aware of our internal programming and learn to deprogram ourselves. Meditation is not programming the mind with thoughts and beliefs or the patterned, repetitious behavior of practices. Rather, it is *seeing*; it is the opening of insight, perception, and understanding. This insight into meditation permeates oneself, inside and out, in all arenas of living.

It opens the possibility of seeing and being touched by the sacred, miraculous intelligence that is life, that is the universe.

## Useful Meditation Practices

In the context of this broader understanding and vision we have been exploring, meditation techniques take their proper place as tools we may choose to use when we are served by them. Several useful meditation tools are offered here.

### Sitting Meditation—"Don't Just Do Something, Sit There"

Sitting is the most commonly practiced mode of formal meditation technique. Our daily lives tend to be filled with activity, even the passive activity of entertainment, television, and reading. Having a formal sitting practice acknowledges the importance and balance of silence and recognizes that some inner domains and inner states of awareness are accessible only by silent entry, when one is very still and inwardly attentive. A Zen master was once asked, "What is meditation?" He replied, "Just sit." That was the extent of the instruction. Sitting is its own reward. In sitting meditation we learn about stillness, and the nature of the mind and thought. We learn to watch and learn from inner processes, and there are many deeper, even unconscious benefits. Sitting helps balance our constant activity and validates the inner journey. A good deal of current scientific research has shown tangible physical and psychological benefits of sitting meditation. After even a short period of sitting, we usually emerge less irritable, more relaxed, and more peaceful. We often find answers to problems or questions, without having consciously thought about them. Sitting meditation seems to bring an ordering of mind. Our culture has an excess of doing and a poverty of being. We could do with a lot more self-reflection, but to the conditioned Western mind the concept of inactivity is seen as wasteful. "Don't just sit there, do something!" is all too familiar.

Sitting meditation teaches us the other side of the coin: "Don't just do something, sit there."

We need not use complicated techniques, nor do we need expensive initiations to access sitting meditation. A practice can simply involve sitting and watching the breath, gazing at a candle flame, or watching the inner landscape. Or it can be as simple as slowing down and taking notice of a moment in the journey. The simplest practices are often the most effective. Find a comfortable sitting position for the body. Most meditators prefer a cross-legged position on a mat on the floor with a pillow or folded blanket under the hips to elevate them four to eight inches. Elevating the hips makes sitting easier and helps to keep the spine straight. If you are not able to sit comfortably on the floor, use the edge of a chair. It is better not to support the back by leaning on a wall or chair back because, when leaning back or reclining, the tendency to fall asleep is greater. Similarly, it is preferable not to lie down for meditation—you will fall asleep more easily. Sitting with a straight back aids awareness and attention and is good for the spine. After getting comfortable, relax the body, take a few deep breaths, and allow a feeling of stillness to arise as you move into your period of sitting. I am reminded of a quick story pertinent to this point in the instruction: After sitting several minutes, a young student leaned over to an old master sitting next to him, and asked, "Okay, now what?" The old man replied, "Nothing, this is it!"

From this point, sitting practice can take several directions. Your only task is to keep attention inward and begin what is called *witness consciousness*—simply witness or watch whatever is happening inside, without trying to change or control it. Watch thoughts and feelings arise and subside. The thoughts will try to grab you and get you involved. Sometimes, until you notice it, you will have boarded a thought train and ridden it to another destination. However, as soon as you see that, come back to your center and the practice of just sitting, just watching.

Try not to control yourself or your mind beyond sitting quietly and watching. You are not trying to *shut up*. The only thing to do is let your body become still, let your breath become still, let your eyes become still, and let whatever unfolds, unfold. There may be thoughts about how you are wasting time, about how noisy the mind is, about whether you're doing it right, and many, many more similar concerns.

At some point—after a few, or even many, meditation sessions—the realization might come that you are not always conscious of all levels involved in this process. This is because the conscious mind cannot plumb the depths of meditation. You will see the results of the practice, though; you will see tracks of it in your life, such as more peace, clarity, and understanding. Be very careful not to fight with your mind or try to force stillness during your sitting meditation. Effort prevents results. That part of the mind that tries to enforce quiet is actually the same part that is chattering. You can only stop the battling process, and the resistance caused by fighting to control thought, by seeing that this battle is futile and giving it up. The mind cannot be stopped by battling. You are the battle.

Sitting practice cannot be done incorrectly. Anything that happens is part of it. There are no disturbances. Any noise, thoughts or distractions become part of the process. Sitting meditation can be a wonderful balm for the mind and nervous system. You can learn about the nature and dynamics of thought. You can learn to release stress, calm the mind, and improve concentration. Too much sitting practice or regimentation, however, can also dull the mind, so be watchful. Find your own rhythms and the amount of practice right for you. This may be every day for a period of time or simply a spontaneous practice. It can be good to try a daily practice for a period of time to learn about the effects and results of sitting. Many people find great benefit in maintaining a daily sitting meditation practice.

## Breath Meditation

Another form of sitting practice focuses meditation on the breath. Using the same guidelines above, sit for meditation and put your attention on your breathing. As noted in our discussion of pranayama, it is very difficult to observe the breath without influencing it. Respiration dances on the threshold of the conscious and unconscious. Any attention to breath brings it right back to conscious control. In breathing meditation, simply watch the breath as it moves into inhalation and exhalation and observe any pauses in between. Listen to the sound of the breath and feel its life force.

After some minutes, your breathing may slow and deepen and become quieter. You may begin to flow with the natural rhythms and movements of breath and life. Sometimes the breath may stop for a time. Control of inhalations and exhalations will fade as you watch the breath breathe itself. If attention wanders or lapses, simply bring it back again. Breath meditation is very relaxing and it soothes the nervous system.

## Candle Meditation

Fire has been part of ceremony since ancient times. Yogis see fire as a portal or doorway to other dimensions and perceptions. Fire exists on the threshold between the tangible physical world and the invisible world of energy and waves. Fire purifies and reduces things to their essential components. Flames have both form and formlessness, and they contain the three primal elements—darkness (smoke, ash, and the dark center of the flame), heat (perceived as motion and energy), and light. Meditation on a flame can bring mystical, spiritual, and religious feeling. Even a single candle flame exudes golden light and beauty. The flame demonstrates stillness in action. When we gaze on a flame in a windless place while sitting quietly with soft breathing, the flame appears to become completely still and unmoving, but it is actually full of great energy and motion. Like a held asana, it is another of nature's standing waves.

The flame has been a great teacher to yogis since ancient times. Even a small candle flame is connected to the sacred fires of all times. Fire teaches us about the circle of life from light and energy, to matter and plant, and back to sound and light.

Candle gazing, called *tratakum* in Sanskrit, can be practiced in the light or in the dark; however, a darkened room is usually preferable. Place a candle at or near eye level and come into sitting meditation position. Gaze at the candle steadily with open or half-open eyes, absorbing yourself in all aspects of the nature of the flame. Naturally, after a time, your eyes will close. You can visualize or feel the presence of the flame within and sometimes you may even continue to see it inwardly. Spend a period of time in the healing, transformational energy of fire.

## Sound and Music

Sound and music are integral parts of meditation. The yoga tradition includes unique practices of using pure sound structures for concentration and meditation. The most common is meditation on the ancient, primordial sound OM. We hear the sound of OM in the wind, the ocean, or even in the din of a crowd or traffic. As a syllable, OM refers to everything, and to nothing; it has no specific meaning but points to all things and to their source. Chanting OM alone or in a group harmonizes and aligns many subtle vibrational frequencies.

Listening to good music nourishes the soul. Music is one of the most important changers and movers of consciousness, and it is a powerful conveyer of evolutionary information. Sound and music reach layers and levels of resonance and communication not possible through other forms of expression. Music plays an important role in a broad definition of meditation and should be included in any discussion of it. We usually think of meditation in terms of silence, but sound and music are also portals to different dimensions of consciousness. Listening to potent music can become a meditation in and of itself, as important as sitting in silence.

## Mantra Meditation

A common form of meditation involves using a mechanical tool like a *mantra*—a sound, syllable, or phrase that is repeated during the meditation practice. Popular mantras include OM, of course, and *ram, shanti,* and *soham*—and there are thousands more. The practice usually involves sitting quietly for a period of time and saying the mantra silently and mentally, sometimes using mala or a rosary. Repeating mantras can calm the mind and have beneficial physiological and psychological benefits. The practice is not hard to learn. Simply sitting and repeating OM silently for a period of time calms the mind and body and gives other benefits.

Unfortunately, a lot of magic and superstition often accompanies some mantra practices. Mantra repetition is one of the oldest forms of mind control. Mantras can be used to calm and control the mind, but also can subject a person to another's control. A mantra cannot be repeated without also unwittingly strengthening the belief system conveyed with and surrounding that mantra. Following the prescription for repetition implies the acceptance of the associated beliefs about the power of the mantra and the importance of its use. We can get high, feel good, and get benefits from mantra repetition, but like any tool, it cuts both ways and can also detrimentally program us to become mechanical, dull, and repetitive. Overuse of mantra can also lead to inability to *stop* repeating the mantra in the same way that singing a song or jingle too much gets it stuck in our head. I am not saying not to experiment with or use mantra meditation. It can be beneficial if practiced wisely, attentively, and judiciously.

## Body Meditation

Hatha yoga philosophy frames our work, practice, and experience in the body as essential parts of meditation. Human life and the human body express the greatest of life's miracles. The vast intelligence of the universe presents itself microcosmically in the body. As a complete and sophisticated system of physical culture, Hatha yoga is a meditation in and of itself. Caring for the body, learning to listen to the body's intelligence and feedback, and watching the body's cycles through the months and years is part of meditation. Asana practice creates the ever illuminative process of constant learning from the psychophysical intelligence and life force. Hatha yogis know that yoga practice restores deep levels of balance and energy and constitutes an integral part of meditation and spiritual awareness.

## Self-Study

*Swadhyaya,* which means study of self, or meditation on oneself, is part of the fullness of meditation. Swadhyaya refers to self-watchfulness, self-awareness, and also to the study of illuminating writings or texts. Self-study, watching and learning about the self, is another form of meditation. Studying and meditating on oneself should not become the stiff, contrived behavior of self-consciousness, but remain a dynamic process of seeing and learning.

## Solitude

We may observe that birds landing on a long wire place themselves with perfect spacing—each bird allowing the personal space to spread wings and fly. This observation offers a valuable lesson about each person's need for space and freedom. Yogis have long emphasized the value of taking some personal, alone time to recharge, center, and reconnect with our own essence. Solitude includes personal, silent time. Some lessons are only learned in silence and silence is a lesson in itself. Solitude is balanced by *satsanga,* or gathering with the wise, which implies spending time, and cross-pollinating, in community with other yogis to trade ideas, opinions, and insights.

## Relationship

Meditation is usually viewed as a solitary practice, a movement within. A yogi I met said, "You know, we're all saints when we're alone. It is much easier to be saintly when you're by yourself, when there is no one to rub up against. We need relationship to discover our true selves and to see how we're doing." We cannot see all of ourselves without a mirror, a reflection. Relationship and daily life offer that reflection. The mirror of relationship reflects and reveals parts of us to ourselves. Relationship is the dance of control and surrender in the balance and discovery of love, cooperation, creation, and mutual reflection. Our relationships define us in context—with family, friends, loved ones, society, the world, with the planet, and with all things. When more of us learn to see and operate from this perception, we will create a different, better world.

## The Spirituality of Nature

> Look deep, deep into nature and then you'll
> understand everything better.
>
> ALBERT EINSTEIN

Any definition of meditation, any spiritual perspective, that does not hold within it the importance of communion, attunement, and learning from nature seriously lacks perspective. Nature is the ultimate healer and the powerful balancer of energy. Communion with nature is a key part of enlightened living—the essence of the wholeness of living. Sitting by a waterfall, by a river or the sea, by a tree, under the stars or the moon, facing the sunrise or sunset—all these are as much a part of meditation as anything else. A solitary walk in a beautiful, natural place (an opportunity becoming tragically limited) is the perfect ingredient for wellness, joy, and insight. We cannot say where or how deep insights or revelations might occur. They are as likely to take place in nature as on the meditation cushion.

Practitioners who spend far too many hours in temples and darkened rooms practicing control or mental repetition frequently neglect nature meditation. This is not meant to demean the inner journey and experience. Inner visionary experience can be divinely magical, immeasurably beautiful, enrapturing and mystical. The inner visionary experience allows us to see into many dimensions, through biochemical and mystical doorways penetrating into the many layers of consciousness. These perceptions can take us to the place where the line between physical and nonphysical, even between this dimension and another, between life and death, cannot be drawn with certainty. But the outer world of nature and the cosmos are of the same infinite, intricate order and offer the same level of perceptual experience.

We too often move through life without tuning into the world of natural beauty and power all around us. Are we in tune with the cycles of the moon, tides, wind, and weather? We spend so much time in environments where we control the temperature, the light, the sounds, even thought. Nature is too easily framed as another source of entertainment. People often go to forests and rivers in the same way they go to amusement parks. They look at the trees, have some fun, take a few photos—but have they learned how to commune deeply?

We cannot exist without nature—in fact, we *are* nature. We breathe in the oxygen that the trees and plants exhale. We exhale carbon dioxide and the world of plants breathes it in. We eat the gifts of the plant kingdom and give back fertilizer. In fact, the magic of photosynthesis from matter, light, and cosmic energy *is* the source of all life. The light of the sun feeds and illuminates the earth, and helps form the clouds that travel the planet bringing the rains, creating the lakes and rivers. The water we drink is made of cloud and sun. Therefore, the body is made up of earth, sun, clouds, and rivers. In our solar system, the Sun and planet Earth are smoldering stardust, still hot at the core. So it is not only poetic to say we are the stars, we are the rivers, we are the sun, we are the earth. We have the opportunity to see and live in this harmonious perception. Seeing this *is* meditation, and not just *a* meditation. We need not sit in our rooms and mentally repeat "Tat Twam Asi. I am the earth. I am the stars. I am the trees." That is only thought and thinking. We can see this circle of life, this living organism of which we are a part, through communion with nature. We learn the nature of balance by going into the balance of nature.

The wonderful book *Siddhartha,* by Herman Hesse,[6] illustrates the power of nature to heal and enlighten. Siddhartha spends his life in search of spirituality and self-knowledge. He becomes a mendicant wanderer, studies with every manner of teacher, does extreme ascetic practices, fasts till near death, and becomes a yogi. Finally, he quits the ascetic life and becomes a wealthy businessman. In his old age he goes to live with a boatman with whom he crossed a river many times. In the end he finds self-realization and enlightenment by giving up the search, communing with the river of life, and watching the river flow.

We spend most of our time living in worlds of our own thought and creation—cities, houses, cars, ideas, conversations, thinking are all our own creations. But nature is not our creation—it *is* creation. When in nature, we are in creation itself. Even a short time by rivers or trees, or spending time in a park, or sitting in the light of the moon, leaves one more whole and recharged. The wind is our breath, the water our circulation, the mountains and stones our bones, and the plants our skin. We can often learn more from a tree, the wind, or the sea than from authorities or volumes on meditation. The earth is an organism. Every plant, person, animal, and river is part of the balance. We are not here to renounce the earth but to learn from it and take care of it. And we must remember, in all of our arrogance about taking care of the earth, that actually it is the earth that is taking care of us. The only compassionate, intelligent, and loving response is to do the same in turn. This is the vision we need to operate from. When more of us have this understanding, we will stop destroying our home.

Another of the great lessons we can learn from nature is that change, growth, and evolution occur through errors and mistakes. When we are not afraid of error, we are more open to growth and our past mistakes transform into the stepping stones of future success and deeper understanding.

The inward journey seeks the god, *within;* the outward journey finds god and goddess, *without.* Divinity exists in the outer world; it is all around us. Divine energy flows in the ever blossoming, eternal present of nature. Every corner of nature emanates that sacredness we seek in our rituals, beliefs, and practices. Nature's teaching is immediate, ever present, and infinite. We are totally immersed in the infinity of nature, the nature of the earth, and of the cosmos. It is beginningless and endless. The one and the many, unity and diversity, reflect and create each other in the same way matter and energy are one and the same. Entering into deep communion and connection with nature, which is not of human creation but *is* creation, is one of the integral parts of whole living, meditation, and spirituality.

## Soma, Nectar of the Gods

No exploration into yoga and meditation would be complete without a look at the ancient lineage of sacred plants and herbs that, many assert, are at the origins of religious experience and spirituality. We live in a time of drug hysteria that calls for a more intelligent understanding that doesn't lump every psychoactive substance, plant, or herb into the category of dark and dangerous. *Soma* was an ancient brew or drink prepared by sages and yogis that was said to bestow health, strength, insight, spiritual visionary experience, and communion with divinity. This sacred drink, also called *amrita* or nectar of the gods, opened the mind, heart, and inner landscape while purifying and healing the body. The word *amrita* means nectar. It comes from the word *mrita,* which means death, and the addition of the *a-* to make *a-mrita,* which thus means nondeath or immortality. Soma use dates back to the ancient time of the Vedas and origins of yoga.

Researchers have suggested that soma was made from psychoactive mushrooms or possibly from a combination of plants, like the Middle Eastern *haoma,* or Syrian Rue, and various herbs. The formula and exact nature of this "nectar of immortality" has been lost, possibly forever, in the mists of antiquity. The Amazon region holds what is probably a similar sacred brew, called *ayahuasca,* which means vine of the souls or vine of the dead. For centuries, and probably thousands of years, such plant admixtures have played a primary role in indigenous people's spirituality, healing, and their discovery of a vast pharmacy of medicines and healing herbs. We owe much of our pharmacopeia to the legacy from indigenous peoples, their sacramental practices, and great knowledge of medicinal plants.

I touch on the topic of plant sacraments because it is a timely subject and something I am repeatedly asked about. I was very fortunate, early in my studies of yoga and mysticism, to have had the opportunity to meet and practice with researchers and explorers of the soma tradition and other entheogens. It is important to realize that there is a right place and proper use for everything. Plant intelligence has informed human consciousness since the beginning of time. We are dependent on plants and live in symbiotic relationship with them. To make certain plants illegal is ignorance. Rather, we need to learn their language, receive their gifts, and learn the right and intelligent use of all things. As Paracelsus, an alchemist and a founder of modern medicine, stated, "The difference between a poison and a medicine is dosage."

There are neural pathways in the brain that are more ancient than our beliefs, philosophies, and religious proscriptions. There are keys to the doorways of the rich interior landscape that open dimensions of beauty, order, intelligence, immense complexity, and sacredness beyond measure. These realities can be so powerful, brilliant, and intense that, while visiting them, our world seems like a distant hallucination, in the way that these other realities can seem hallucinatory from this one. Seeing and being touched by these mystical experiences can change us and help us in positive ways with insights into self-healing, enlightened living, and the wholeness of life. Our bodies and brains operate on chemical messengers and information exchange systems in nature. Some scholars and evidence show that medicinal plants were probably at the origin of religious and mystical experience. To say plant sacraments are unnatural, and that practices, rituals, and belief systems created by man are natural, is an absurdity. It is a shame that fear and conditioning can preclude the greatest journey . . . within.

> *Soma, soma, devamritam, parama jyoti, namo, namah.*
> "To soma, nectar of the gods, who reveals the divine light, salutations, again salutations." I quietly offered this ancient chant as we floated down the jungle river hanging in hammocks. The Amazon reflected the night as lightning bugs lit the sky opening up mysteries of the cosmos, revealing beatific sights in holographic worlds of light, intricacy, and geometric, oscillating wonder. We were drifting in and beholding the matrix of life. We floated into a void of darkness that took shape and form, turning into corridors of color, opening into the field of dreams. All my relations, the sweat lodge prayer of Native Americans, took on new meaning as each relationship in life paraded before me, viewed with the lens of insight from the sacred vine.

There are keys to the doorways of mind and consciousness that are guarded by phantom demons of fear and certainty. They bring dread to the brittle-minded and self-righteous, preventing entry. These demons may guard the entrance but the reward inside, ironically, is the gift of responsibility and the wisdom of uncertainty.

**Astronomical or Science Meditation**

Personal mystical experience, and the experience of Oneness and the interconnectedness of all things can occur spontaneously, and through meditation, drumming, shamanic practices, plant teachers, from fasting, near-death experiences, and from communion with nature. This Oneness experience also seems to be accessible from meditation on the cosmos, through deep contemplation of astronomical and scientific principles. The Oneness experience becomes a deep foundation and field of reference that informs and fills our hearts and consciousness with the infinite, the source of all. Both religious and scientific inquiry can take us to the infinite reaches of the universe where the individual self dissolves.

We can learn to raise our awareness, perspective, and frame of reference to cosmic proportions. Allowing consciousness to move out toward the vast perspective of galactic and intergalactic proportions, and into the relationships of matter, high-energy particles, white holes, and black holes of immeasurably large numbers has a profound effect on consciousness. Viewed from the cosmic perspective, the human frame of reference is nearly infinitesimal in comparison, almost illusory in that vast sea of time and space. We can access this vision by gazing at the stars, the Milky Way, and out into the mysterious universe. We can also access it by contemplation of cosmic proportions. The beauties and revelations of science provide an extraordinary meditation journey. A few of these numbers are offered here.

It took many centuries for humanity to learn more about the nature, size, and scope of even our tiny corner of the universe. For millennia we assumed that the planet Earth was the center of an unchanging universe. It was only in 1609 that Galileo invented the telescope. Now we have learned and seen the vastness of our galactic home. Let your mind take the astronomer's and mathematician's journey.

Light travels at a speed of 12 million miles a *minute* and now we know that the nearest stars lie 5 light *years,* or 31,500,000,000,000 miles away! This distance would require approximately a 100,000-year journey in today's spacecraft. Our Milky Way spiral galaxy consists of 100 billion stars. Think about that for a moment. Galaxies are composed of countless numbers of stars. Our galaxy is enormous beyond conception but it is only a part of clusters of galaxies of astounding size—galaxies that span hundreds of millions of light years across.

Our current science and instruments can see about 15 billion light years. The Milky Way itself is about 10 billion years old with millions of stars forming and dying all the time. Supernovas create components of life, such as oxygen, gas, and the elements. Earth itself is truly stardust, a speck of our galactic center cooling off. Aside from these vast cosmic distances with black holes, white holes, supernovas, and star systems, there is the microcosmos with quarks, protons, neutrons, neutrinos, and possibly antimatter.

Gases, rain, radiation, and bombarding cosmic elements shaped Earth. Our planet revolves around the Sun at 900 miles per hour. The stars move away a million miles a day at about 40,000 miles per hour. The outer spiral arm of the Milky Way galaxy, where Earth resides, is 100,000 light years wide. Our galaxy is only one of hundreds of billions of galaxies, many of which are far larger.

If we lived the entire history of the earth in one hour, in the first 50 minutes we would be in a world of single-cell organisms. Animal life existed only in the last ten minutes, and all of human history would have occurred in the last one-hundredth of a second of that hour.

Our Earth actually exists on an energy-matter, space-time continuum: From our galactic Milky Way center, our energy source, through time and space, through the creation of all the elements of the physical universe, from cosmic energy and radiation, to light; and then coalescing down to the creation of every molecule and element on this speck of stardust called Earth, which is bathed in the light of the sun and the radiation from the galaxy, and on which self-reflecting humans were born to marvel at the wonder of it all.

We have no way to understand truly these massive numbers, times, and distances—and that is the point. Contemplating the vastness of the universe can be a catalyst for transcending the normal limits of consciousness. When we actually hold these perspectives in awareness, they become a dissolving and illuminating, transformational perception of the immeasurable. This vision becomes a form of cosmic consciousness. Whenever you have the opportunity, on a starlit night, lie back, meditate on the cosmos, and take yourself on that cosmic voyage.

## Death Meditation

Meditation on death can open our hearts and fill us with love and compassion. Thinking about our own death can, after moving through the fear, lead to cherishing each moment we have. We don't like to think about death, and we usually push the idea of our own end into the distant future. But death is ever present, all around us, and even sits on our shoulder. The word yoga means, and reminds us about, connection and reintegration. Death teaches us about the inevitability of separation, ending, and that all things must pass.

On my first trip to India, a yogi took me to the funeral pyres near a river. Cremation is very common in India and some yogis even make a meditation practice of watching the fires and burning bodies. My yogi friend suggested we try to watch a burning body, crackling and charring as it disappears into its essence of dust and light. To our Western mindset and conditioning, this practice may seem macabre, even diabolical. But in the East, the death meditation is often seen as a way of awakening us to our ephemeral nature and opening our hearts to care and love. We do not emphasize this aspect of death, nor talk about it much in our culture, but we have similar experiences. When we attend a funeral of a loved one, we usually leave with a full heart, more sensitive to others and more caring. I remember making a call to my aging father, who was normally a bit stiff and self-absorbed, and finding him unusually open and caring. He asked a lot of questions about how I was doing and how my life was going. Sensing how differently he was behaving, I asked him if anything unusual or important had happened. He said no. I asked what he did that day and he said he visited my mother's grave at the cemetery and had been looking over arrangements he had made for his own burial plot next to her. I realized that my father was doing the death meditation and that it had opened his heart.

As I watched that body burn on a pile of logs by the River Ganga, my horror and revulsion slowly began to subside. My heart began to soften and open and I saw deeper into life and death through the doorway of flames. We sat by the sacred river and watched the body melt away into a film of ash floating downstream. In the evening light, long clouds lined the sky. There was sadness and joy, ending and beginning. An extraordinary stillness and beauty filled the night with the pink glow against the blue sky reflecting and enhancing the delicate, green spring grasses lining the hills. Slowly the light, and with it the beauty, faded and I almost began to mourn its brevity and departure, as we do the inevitable loss of things dear. But the moonlight arrived and began to light the skies, trees, and clouds. Beauty began revealing itself, reborn again in new ways. We can mourn the loss of the past or keep our eyes on the ever-present, constantly changing dance of dissolution and creation.

## Looking Forward, Looking Backward

Another form of meditation or contemplation involves one or several sittings, during which we try to project and experience self in old age, near the end of life. The meditator visualizes him- or herself with diminished capacities and abilities, such as much less energy, mobility, and eyesight, and imagines the other unpleasant qualities of old age. Why do such a seemingly depressing exercise? Because it is a common folly of youth to feel "these things will never happen to me." In the naiveté of youth, we feel we will overcome the problems of sickness and old age.

We will practice yoga, we will eat properly, and learn to heal ourselves. Fortunately, we can preserve our vitality to a great extent, but bodies do wear out and age. The body is not a perpetual motion machine. Other than the universe and life itself, perpetual, eternal machines do not exist. The realization that these things could happen to us offers a source of wisdom, and like the death meditation, this awareness can inform life, infusing it with appreciation, care and attention, and awareness of life's preciousness.

This contemplation is not a negative approach, but actually the seed of something positive and illuminating. When the Buddha was born into a royal family, an astrologer advised his father that this new son would either become a great king or a great monk. Fearing that his son might leave the kingdom, the father brought him up isolated from exposure to sickness, old age, and death. When he got older, the Buddha toured his kingdom, and saw the sick, aged, and dying for the first time. He was powerfully thrown into this meditation and it eventually led him to his own awakening and the discoveries he went on to share and teach.

## How Much to Practice

All of these forms of meditation practice can be beneficial and enjoyable, and can be used in any combination. Opportunities for them abound. There are no formulas on how much or how often to use them. They offer an ongoing journey of experimentation, practice, and learning from experience.

After several years of traditional yoga study and practice, I had the opportunity to travel in India and Europe with a bright, unconventional yogi. He encouraged and enjoyed *vichara*—the process of deep inquiry, questioning, and discussion. At that time I was still very steeped in traditional thinking, and I believed meditation must be structured and practiced daily as part of one's routine. The yogi, who led meditation classes, kept taking the opposite viewpoint, emphasizing the spontaneity and freedom of real meditation. After a couple of days of debate, I finally began to see his perspective on meditation as something that has to occur naturally without contrived effort. I began to feel free, and excited, letting go of effort. I got up, and as I was leaving the room, I said, "Thank you very much. I feel very freed up and now see meditation as something that occurs naturally, a *happening.*" As I was closing the door, he smiled and said, "One more thing, Ganga. Be sure to let it happen regularly!" Now that he had swung me the other way, he was sure to get in the last blow. Both sides of the argument have their validity. There is a need and benefit of learning control and there is also that which is beyond control.

Meditation balances an interplay of control and surrender, faith and questioning, reverence and self-empowerment. It is selflessness balanced by individuality, or *self-fullness.* It requires holding firmly and letting go. It brings grace and harmony. It perceives the miraculous and the sacred. Meditation is all of life, the wholeness of life, the ending of time, and the essence of yoga.

## CHAPTER 10

# Spirituality, Enlightenment, and the Miraculous

seeker of truth
follow no path
all paths lead where
truth is here

E.E. CUMMINGS

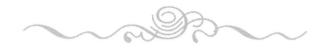

Our deeply rooted concepts of spirituality developed over millennia in religious traditions from around the world that had their beginnings ages ago in times when human consciousness and the state of our knowledge were very different from what they are today. Tradition was a necessary means of passing knowledge from generation to generation. Strong controls on society were needed, since survival depended on generations living as their ancestors had taught. Centuries, even millennia, may have passed with little or no profound change in traditions. Memory, custom, and repetition were requisite for the survival and maintenance of societies and cultures without books, tape systems, computers, and other mechanisms of mass information storage and distribution. The advent of science and technology introduced huge challenges that upset the ancient equilibrium of religious thought and culture. Science allowed many inexplicable and seemingly miraculous things to be proved, explained, demonstrated, and acted upon while creating many new miracles beyond even those reported by religion. There are legends, for example, of yogis levitating or hovering above the ground, but now we can "levitate" hundreds of people at once across the seas at thirty-five thousand feet.

## Our Relation to the One

We now live in a very different world. There are many beautiful principles and gems of wisdom in ancient religion, but human knowledge has grown exponentially. Given the many insights and advances in our culture, many of the ancient beliefs, practices, and philosophies no longer seem appropriate or consonant with broader, modern perspectives. Much Eastern philosophy grew from the explanations and teachings of mystics who claimed experiences of divinity, or of the Oneness of the universe. The core belief in this perspective is that the underlying truth and reality in life is the One, and that the everyday world of diversity and individuality in which we live is actually an illusion, called *maya*. Worldly existence is often regarded merely as a means for getting us back to union with the One, with God, or to enlightenment. Thought, ego, self-centeredness, desire, and attachment are usually defined in these traditions as obstacles to be eliminated in order to go beyond separateness into Oneness and reintegration. While this common yogic perspective has given us many useful insights and transformational practices, it can also be a limiting, *one*-sided perspective.

Seeing Oneness as the only essential true reality can lead to a devaluing of the earth, of life, and personal relationships. In this perspective, our relationship to the transcendent, to the mystical, or to the Teacher, the Guru, is often put above our closest personal relationships, even that with our children. (For example, the Buddha and many other spiritual exemplars are reputed to have left their wives and children to pursue their personal goals of enlightenment.) In fact, a healthy and balanced amount of desire, attachment, and even ego, can be shown to be necessary, inseparable aspects of life with purpose and use. Eastern thought often defines these aspects of life essentially as the obstacles to enlightenment, but it may be wiser to learn to live intelligently with these inherent dimensions of ourselves rather than try to annihilate them. Every living organism, arguably even every physical element and atom, by definition, needs self-defining, self-protective characteristics. Both boundary and permeability are necessary in the universe. We need to understand unity and interconnection, and to value diversity.

## Oneness and the Loss of Diversity

One of the greatest tragedies of modern times is the accelerating loss of diversity, both in nature and culture. We seem to be homogenizing our planet into a oneness of asphalt, TV, and global franchises. This disturbing trend was driven home to me on a journey deep into the Brazilian Amazon with some forest dwellers and shamans.

We had outfitted and taken a boat along a marvelous, snaking river. Two days into the dense jungle, we tied the boat at the river bank and hiked into the forest to see the animals among enormous, ancient trees and vines. It was extraordinarily hot and humid, and after a couple hours of trekking we were all very thirsty and hungry. Suddenly, a loud roar shook the ground. I expected a fleet of army helicopters to pass over but the source was huge, black clouds, which quickly passed overhead with exploding thunder and lightening. The cloud bank began to pour relentless torrents of rain and we were immediately drenched. We only had to cup hands to fill them and drink as if from a faucet.

We ran through the woods, looking for shelter, and came upon a very small village of shabby wooden huts with thatched roofs. Beautiful, smiling children ran to greet us and welcome us into their home. They served us dried coconut and banana and we threw the scraps to their chickens. As I was standing in their living area, I heard some strange, garbled sounds coming out of the next room. I poked my head through the door and was astonished to see a small, old television set with our jungle friends seated around it, watching *Dallas*. I looked outside and saw a small power line and cable line strung through the primeval forest we came to honor. Our modern lifestyle is consuming our ecosphere and also our *ethnosphere*—the diversity of ethnic cultures and wisdom.

The greatest terrorism of our time is the terrorism against our environment—the effects and loss are not only immediate, but will last for generations to come. It is not only a disgrace to lose this diversity, and the unique beauty of different cultures and different parts of the earth, but the earth cannot support a just and equitable distribution of resources at the levels at which we are living in North America.

Diversity is the fabric of life. In the same way that matter and energy are part of one continuum, the One and the Many are a natural, mutually embedded polarity in the universe. In fact, they are necessary counterparts of each other. Diversity is as sacred as unity—the many as relevant, important, and sacred as the One or God. In fact, neither could exist without the other. This perspective can be positive and freeing. Both science and religious mysticism offer insights and pieces of the puzzle of existence. There are many gems and gifts from the past and the understanding and insights presented in this work would not be possible without our ancestors and traditions. While we honor their contributions and their place in the past, it is also the moment to step beyond them. Thousands of years of these ancient ways have brought us to this critical point in our history. Now is the time for something new, a new awakening, a new vision, a new liberation.

## Spirituality Beyond Belief

We need to look at our many long-held beliefs and dogmas to shed new light and to awaken a new perception, a new insight, and a new paradigm of spirituality that better bridges science, technology, and religion, and that stops the degradation of the earth and society. This is more important now than ever before because on many fronts our destructive powers have become global, threatening life as we know it.

Spirituality, and our relationship to it, must change and grow. Spirituality is an evolving, immeasurable energy that is not fixed in definitions, descriptions, and pathways defined for all time thousands of years ago, by cultures without science-based knowledge we now take for granted—biology, astronomy, psychology, archeology, geology, anthropology, quantum physics, evolution, and the many other remarkable discoveries of our times. Right here and now in this new millennium we have the possibility of standing on the shoulders of the past in order to see farther and deeper than humans have seen before. We can open the doorway into lives of exciting adventure, sharing this extraordinary moment in history.

Spirituality and self-realization rest at the core and essence of yoga philosophy. Many people come to yoga primarily for fitness, physical health, and well-being, but even among this group there is often interest and appreciation for the holistic and deeper aspects of yoga. Any exploration into yoga would be incomplete without an inquiry and examination of its spiritual essence. While there is a lot of interest in spirituality among students of yoga, there is often a lack of clarity and understanding. Roughly two broad categories distinguish viewpoints on spirituality. As we have discussed in the area of meditation, one viewpoint is that there is an eternal, spiritual path that has been mapped, discovered, and revealed. This viewpoint assumes we must follow that path as defined by its practices, rituals, and beliefs. The other viewpoint defines spirit and spirituality in a more relativistic manner, seeing spirituality as living and evolving. The first perspective describes spirituality more in terms of specific beliefs, rituals, and defined behaviors, while the second perspective sees the approach to spirituality requiring flexible, living awareness and attunement in order to move and flow with spirit.

Looking at music as an example may help us understand the evolutionary nature of spirituality. Music is not the same as it was when it was first developed. Early forms of music were very limited in range, pitch, and complexity, with simple rhythms and fewer possibilities of instrumentation. Over the centuries music has evolved into many genres and highly complex symphonies that communicate broad ranges of feeling, emotion, and meaning. Similarly, our understanding of spirituality needs to grow and evolve beyond the limits of tradition and ancient mappings.

Spiritual practices are often seen as the essential core that defines and measures spirituality, but it may be wiser and more useful to hold spiritual practices in a similar way that we might hold medicines, and treat ritual, custom, and belief as things to learn the appropriate need and use for on an individual and relative basis. Certain medicines might be very useful to a particular person at particular times but unhelpful or adverse other times. Too often spiritual practices are promoted like snake oils—the cure for all our ills. We may have and need spiritual practice and we must also keep open the possibility of freedom in the way we hold and use them. A free context will keep us open to the awareness and revelations that can only come spontaneously and uninvited, in unstructured, timeless moments. A growing number of yogis see life, not as following a specified path, but rather as a journey into untold possibility. This unfolding understanding requires a constant vigilance of awareness and sensitivity that responds to the moment, guiding us on our way through life's changing seas.

Spirituality is not simply a mechanical process and not something finally obtained or acquired. Important elements contribute to spirituality, such as ethical behavior, right living, right livelihood, caring, and compassion, but the deepest essence lives beyond practices, beliefs, descriptions, and words. It is not advisable to explain or define spirituality with too much detail, and it cannot be captured, owned, or stored up. Ironically, the Sanskrit word for illusion—maya—also means to measure and to define. When we measure and overly structure spirit, we may lose it.

While traveling in the Himalayas, I met many swamis and yogis who seemed caught up in what has come to be called *spiritual materialism*—the concept that spiritual merit can be stored up and accumulated. Some of the swamis seemed condescending to anyone who had not achieved as much as they had. I remember one swami bragging about nearly completing a *puruscharana,* or the repetition of his mantra hundreds of thousands of times. He asked me and others how long we had repeated our mantras; he claimed great wisdom, but he seemed stale and automated. He exemplified spiritual materialism, seeming to see his spirituality as an accounting system in which he had a very good balance sheet. Neither life, wisdom, nor love work like a bank account. Great attainments and lifetimes of merit can evaporate in a moment, and awakening or compassion can come in a flash.

A funny story demonstrates this idea. Once there was a billionaire businessman who had cheated and lied throughout his lifetime to make his fortune. On his death bed, however, he realized his fate and donated his entire estate to charity. When he died, the lords of karma were in a quandary about what to do with his soul. He had done so much evil and had millions of dollars in bad deeds, but because of his gift he ended up ten dollars in the black! The karmic accountants were in a dilemma and appealed directly to God for a decision in this difficult case. God looked over the man's deeds and the balance sheets and replied, "Give him back his ten dollars and tell him to go to Hell!" It is silly to reduce life and spirituality to a measurable system of accounting.

Spirituality can be discovered and touched, and it can touch us, leading to deepening love, insight, and wisdom. It is larger than we are; we exist within it. Our most eloquent words are at best only approximations. Spirituality is like an exquisite flower that blooms when it will. It is not possible to cheapen it so that it can be fully explained or captured in formulated living. It is more like the round, fiery, rising sun peaking through fingers of cloud. Can you convey in words what the sunset is? Even a photograph is a poor approximation. The sunrise can only convey itself.

We may do our sitting practices, our rituals, and mantra repetitions, and become better human beings—or not. History is replete with examples of spiritual practitioners who became or remained tyrants. The message and teaching here is that spirituality cannot be mechanized or automated into systems of practices. Practices have their place, but we must always be vigilant and aware. Spirit is the mysterious, ineffable, flow that reveals itself occasionally in synchronicity, magical moments, and the beauty of perception—as being touched by a sunset or a smile. Synchronicities can be cosmic signposts of the unseen hand of the mysterious and the miraculous. Love is the essence, heart, and the expression of spirituality. Spirituality is the art of living—living with the highest possible excellence, compassion, passion, creativity, artistry, and awe.

We must be careful about organizing and codifying our spirituality. A couple of memorable stories speak to this. In the first, a wise man and his student are walking along the beach. The wise man is instructing his student, who is finally beginning to have flashes of illumination and insight, glimpsing the meaning and depth of life. Following the two men are a devil and his student. The devil's student observes the wise man's student beginning to awaken and is quite nervous and upset. "Do something quickly, master. His student is about to get it!" he says. "Relax, no problem," replies the devil. "Nothing to worry about. After he gets it, all we have to do is help the boy organize it!" Awakening and insight are lost when we apply too much structure and organization. Religion is institutional, spirituality is deeply personal. Direct personal perception that there is no mechanical path to spirituality creates an inner revolution that is the ending of struggle and the awakening of a new energy that is creative and free.

We create similar problems of rigidity by depending on rituals and practices for our spirituality without keeping our eyes and hearts open, as the next story points out. A spiritual seeker spent his life pursuing God, enlightenment, and cosmic consciousness. He lived in monasteries, made pilgrimages, and read all the holy books. In the twilight of his life, he gave up his search and decided to end his days peacefully in the beauty of the mountains and forests. He went deep into the woods and built a camp, where he spent his time in solitude with only the trees, animals, and stars, and eating wild fruits and nuts. Before his death he found peace for the first time, and realized that all his efforts, rituals, and practices seemed more of a hindrance than a help. He found his awakening all around him in life and wanted to share his realization with others but was not strong enough to return to the city where he had lived. So he decided to make a carving that might convey his insight. He cut a tree and carved a beautiful statue of a man with one hand pointing up toward the stars, the other pointing outward toward life; the statue's face was peaceful and smiling. The seeker happened to die one day while sitting in the Lotus position. Many years later, his statue and his bones were found by some pilgrims. They marveled at the bones still resting in the Lotus pose and they pondered the meaning of the statue. "These are the bones of a great yogi," they said. "He left this statue in a mudra of great meaning, and his teachings and this place are obviously very holy." So they built a temple and enshrined the bones and statue. Each day they offered flowers to the carving and sat in the temple to meditate, never seeing the beauty nor the essence toward which it pointed. It is often our habit and mistake to turn living perceptions into ritual and repetitive practice.

We may be living during the time of the birth of a new spirituality. This spirituality is free from restricting dogmas and beliefs that divide. It is deeply connected to the sacredness of the web of life, our planet, and the matrix of symbiotic interrelationships in the diversities all around us. We are all part of that web, that life, that wholeness. Our technologies are here to stay and we must learn to use them properly to serve the well-being of all instead of in service of narrow doctrines, or in service of greed. We need to live and act from a perception of the deepest principles of the interconnectedness and sacredness of life, to see our responsibility to leave our planet better than we found it, and to become more conscious of the consequences of our lifestyles in the near and long term. We could all use a good dose of the ancient principle of *santosha*, or contentment with the pains, joys, and beauties in the simple—but extraordinarily potent—activities of daily life. This spirituality has at its core a new insight, a new awareness, a new consciousness unburdened by limited beliefs, and open to light, love, truth, spirit, and the art of living, choosing the highest levels of action and awareness each moment.

## Evolutionary Enlightenment

Enlightenment is not a place we get to, nor an attainment, but an endless journey of seeing, learning, awakening, and reawakening. Rather than viewing enlightenment as a state of all-knowing perfection, we are better off seeing it as an endless process. It is beyond the scope of this book to go into a comprehensive critique of the enlightenment paradigm, a common spiritual worldview held by yogis that frames final enlightenment as the end, goal, and purpose of life. I am hoping the approaches to personal practice and insight we have explored demonstrate a more dynamic alternative. Rather than viewing enlightenment as a final condition that leaves us in an all-knowing, and often self-righteous, state, it is more valuable to see enlightenment as a continuous, ongoing, ever-changing process—a movement that by nature and necessity must ebb and flow. If our heads are always in the clouds, absorbed in the One, we cannot navigate well among the Many.

In some traditions this *natural,* or temporary, enlightenment is considered a lesser attainment. Is it? What are the implications of considering someone, or considering oneself, to be permanently enlightened? There are no errors for these people; all their deeds and words are in perfect harmony with the universe. Every act is pure love and truth. Being in their presence is seen as a blessing. This is the formula for abuse and megalomania. There are those who may take issue with this perspective and point to perfected ones of the past or present as faultless masters. I suggest being very cautious of such claims or they may become the ultimate seduction. Trust yourself and the development of your own insight.

To oversimplify, it may be spiritual to do what feels good, what serves us and the world, what turns us on, and what improves our wisdom, self-knowledge, understanding, and self-esteem. We can base the practices we choose on these guiding lights, not only on what people say we should do to become whole. The bottom line is each one of us must decide what is right and appropriate for ourselves. We all depend on and learn from each other and from our teachers. Education is the foundation of living, but unquestioning obedience to, and worship of, teachers—long a tradition in India—supports authoritarianism, exploitation, and coercion. We must question our teachers, ourselves, and our beliefs. It has been said, "Don't believe what you think." Thought is fallible and belief is often blind. The word *belief* itself is spelled with *lie* in the middle.

Once in discussion, a wise yogi showed me how holding enlightenment as a goal was a misconception. We were having a lively and profound discussion in which he was leading me into a trap that would free me from this idea. I was questioning him about the nature of enlightenment and obviously I was holding onto the idea of a *final* enlightenment. I kept phrasing my questions with "When you get enlightened ..." or "After you're enlightened ..." My friend kept pushing me and replying, "Yes, WHEN? ... when you get enlightened? Then? Then what?" I struggled with his questions and kept replying in a way that framed enlightenment as an attainment or final goal to reach, after which one would be totally clear and wise. He retorted to my replies until finally he got me to see and realize something and I exclaimed, "Ah ha, you 'get there,' you get enlightened, and think you've arrived, so then you can go back to sleep!" Right in chorus with me, he said, "Then you can go back to sleep!" There was a pregnant silence and then he added that there is no final destination. Thinking one has arrived is darkness once again. He went on to explain further how he saw enlightenment as enlightened living, constantly reawakening and always being alert, questioning, and watchful.

Enlightenment also implies light—light itself. Light comes in many forms—insight, awareness, illumination of the dark corners of our consciousness, illumination of the darkness of our fears and neuroses. Light dispels darkness. Light is also the beauty of nature, both inner and outer. Light can take us on transformational journeys deep inside our own consciousness, revealing countless and immeasurable mysteries and visions of multi-hued, jeweled inner worlds. Light permeates the universe. Even matter is another form of light. All that we see as manifest creation—planets, stars, the sun—are, in a sense, just a part of the smoldering, cooling light energy in the universe. Light illumines our paths and worlds, yet itself remains one of the greatest mysteries.

Enlightenment is the discovery of the sublime, the mystical, and the mysterious. It is seeing connection and separation; it is merging into the interconnectedness of all things. *Interconnectedness* is a good term because it implies both oneness and separation. At deep levels of perception there is neither up nor down, left nor right, neither the experiencer nor the experience. Enlightenment explores and resides at the indefinable edge where life and death meet. It wanders in the mystery of the Divine, beyond the mind of man. But we must also be very careful because enlightenment can become the ultimate driving desire, the cosmic carrot on the end of a stick, pulling us into a life of struggle toward unattainable goals of perfection, purity, and perpetual bliss. Like all things, seasons and cycles come and go. We may have timeless moments of enlightenment, deep insight, revelation, and realization. We may merge into that which is beyond us, into the source that sustains us. Then we must come back down the ladder of consciousness into the daily moments of living. The time of the light, the time of vision and perception, later becomes a distant guiding vision. That light itself lives only in its own moment. When we rely too heavily on past insights and realizations, we may lose the light of perception that lives in the present moment. The enlightenment of today can become the ignorance of tomorrow, if one isn't vigilant.

Part of enlightenment involves lightening up a bit. This does not imply that we should not take things seriously, but that we should see the humor in life and in ourselves. Lightening up also points to the importance of ridding ourselves of some of the mental and psychological baggage we have accumulated. To let go we must also let go of the fear of standing alone—of being without supports or crutches. To move beyond our hopes of being saved by gurus or perfect paths, we must go through our fears. The demons of fear guard the gateways to freedom. When we let go of the weight of enlightenment, as a permanent state of supreme wisdom and all-knowingness—which may be nothing more than an abstraction or concept—we are closer to the possibility of seeing the insight, light, and delight in each moment in the world outside us, and in the infinite worlds within us.

## The Mystery: Death and Time

Death is the greatest mystery and the ultimate unknown. As we have seen, death embraced is a great teacher, a potent meditation, and life is the greatest guru. Living and dying, beginning and ending, are intertwined. Death is part of life's teaching. Yoga, religion, and spirituality concern, at the core, our relationship with death. I use the word *relationship,* instead of *knowledge* or *understanding,* because death has its own life; it is the essence of change and mystery. We cannot completely know death. As we grow older and experience the deaths of loved ones, this relationship with death can bring insight, love, maturity, compassion, and appreciation for our own mortality. Having beliefs in philosophies and hopes about the meaning of death does not inform and enlighten living in the same way that having a relationship with death does—seeing death, change, beginning and ending, in the movement of living.

Seeing the presence of death in life gives life its preciousness. Over millennia philosophers, yogis, and sages have discussed and inquired into the possible limits of understanding death. In mystical experiences, altered states, and meditation, it is possible to experience entire lifetimes, even eternity, in very short spans of time. Many have reported back from these experiences and described feeling they lived vast periods of time in short moments. This points to the elasticity and relativity of mind states and mental time. The concept of the relativity of time appears occasionally in ancient texts such as *The Yoga Vasistha*.[7] A story is told there of the god Vishnu walking and enjoying the beauty of the earth with his student, Narada, who is a wise and advanced student. Narada is in such joy walking with his teacher and wants to understand why people suffer in illusion. He asks Vishnu to please explain the power that time, delusion, and illusion hold over people. Vishnu says it is much too complicated for such a beautiful day and he sits down on a log on a mountain ridge. Their canteens are empty so he asks Narada to please find them some water.

Narada leaves and has to hike a long way before he finds a river. As he is filling the canteens, he sees on the other bank a beautiful young maiden bathing naked in the river. He is entranced by her full breasts, long hair, and shapely legs as he watches her bathe. After she dresses he crosses the river and introduces himself. They are both quite taken with each other and Narada decides to stay awhile. After some days they fall completely in love, and he asks her father for her hand in marriage. They are wed, and have two beautiful children. One day a huge storm arrives, bringing incessant rains. The river swells and starts to wash away the village, with his wife and sons. Narada, in great fear and panic, desperately tries to rescue his family from the rising torrents, but they drown in front of his eyes. He struggles to the banks of the river, barely saving himself, and sits on the shore wailing. Sobbing in overwhelming grief, he feels a tap on his shoulder. It is Vishnu, who says, "Narada, where have you been? It has been two hours since I asked you to fetch us some water!" Narada comes to his senses, looks around, and sees there is no village, no flood. He realizes he has dreamed or experienced a lifetime in a few minutes. Vishnu winks at him with a look that reminds Narada he had asked to see the power of mind and illusion. This story is sometimes used to denigrate sexuality, relationships, and attachments, purporting them to be dream, illusion, and a lower level of reality. But the story also has the subtler message repeated in this old text that time is fluid, mental states are relative, and time can expand and compress in near-death experience, altered states, dream, and reveries. In a flash, time collapses from years to minutes for Narada, and he realizes the pliability of mental time and mental suffering. He sees how in the twinkling of an eye everything can change when life taps us on the shoulder. Life can tap any of us on the shoulder at any moment, and then we can see things in a whole new way.

Science too has shown that time is warped and space is curved. Philosophers have argued that even if people report back from near-death or altered states about having personally experienced reincarnation or other lifetimes, their experience could in fact actually all have occurred in the final moments, the final powering down, of the brain itself. So, even to one who believes in or has experienced reincarnation or the eternity of time in a single moment, a deep, objective inquiry reveals that death remains and veils the great mystery. In death is the force of change and transformation that can come as a gentle wind or a tempest. That is why the mystery of death is given a central role in the spiritual process of moving into deeper awareness and understanding. Desire to understand what lies behind the doorway of death has given birth to religious belief and philosophy.

The doctrine of karma and reincarnation is an attempt to explain this mystery. Reincarnation is central in many Eastern philosophical traditions. We need not overly burden ourselves trying to determine whether this belief is true. If the doctrine of reincarnation is true, then what we do with our present life is of crucial importance. How we live now will determine our future incarnations and potential freedom. However, if this life is our only life, then in the same way, how we live now is again vitally important. If this is our only life, it is our only opportunity. In both viewpoints we are left with the importance of the present moment.

When death remains the mystery uncovered by hope and belief, then joy and presence in the moment take on their rightful significance. Mystery gives life depth and meaning. If we knew everything about our future, life might become boring and lose meaning. In a similar way that explaining a joke or revealing the end of a story or movie can take the life out of them, removing the mystery and uncertainty from life would make living barren. Mystery is immense and cannot be removed. No matter how much we uncover, the mystery still remains. We can only remove our awareness of the immensity of mystery by covering it, and deadening it, with beliefs and certainties. What we want is certainty, but what we have is relativity. There is great beauty in the mystery of life. Part of life is mystery, and remains mysterious, beyond teaching, thought, or explanation.

## Navigating Life

All navigation systems use at least two points of reference. We cannot navigate and find our location, our way, and our destination with only one point of reference. To perceive location and depth, we use two vantage points, such as our two ears and our two eyes. This principle can be applied to navigating through life. For example, there are *heart-centered* people who say that we should listen only to our hearts, and always follow the heart. There are *mind-centered* people who say we should primarily rely on intellect, mind, thought, and brain power to find our way and solve our problems. Why not see that both heart and mind, male and female, control and surrender, and the many other polarities of life are necessary vantage points for reference and navigation? To steer ourselves through the constantly changing experience of life, we need to use the polarity of opposites. We do not live in a black-and-white reality. Black and white may be at the ends of a spectrum of navigation, but the matrix of life and living takes place between in shades of gray and in the multiplicity of nuance of color, shape, and form. The heart is balanced by the head, the head by the heart. Personal intuition is balanced by external knowledge and feedback. Both the One and the Many, our interconnectedness and our individuality, create and reflect each other. Giving different perspectives, these many vantage points guide us and bring our paths into view.

With your own light, enhanced by the light of teachers, friends, and others, you can navigate your life, your meditation, your spirituality. However dim and flickering, your light will grow and begin to illumine that way that is uniquely yours, that only you can discover for yourself. Your own journey can be a constantly enthralling, endlessly fascinating, description-defying movement in the enchantment and mystery of living. *Become a light unto yourself.*

Are you ready for total inner freedom? Can you live free from dependencies on dogmas, beliefs, gurus, churches, and temples? Can you loosen the bondage of your own fixed ideas? This freedom, beyond fear and acceptance, lies across the void of your own failings and ignorance, and lights your own unique path, a path that can never be walked by another. Can you be free from images and spiritually adolescent cosmic fantasy, living in the potent presence of the mysterious and the miraculous, the sacred in all things, seeing the play and constant movement of life and death that is awakening? Can you live beyond images and personifications of the infinite in the freedom, joy, and aliveness of the unknown? These questions have no answers—they are the light on the path.

Meditation and spirituality can be simple and natural, or made into complex forms of mental contortion and inner battle that supposedly take years of effort to master. What is one to do instead? Be quiet, sit, and breathe in a place of beauty or with the simplicity of a candle flame.

Sit under the stars with a quiet mind and no goal. Be attentive to all things in life. Honor yourself. Laugh at yourself. Listen to the voice of your own body. Carry joy and light on your path. Listen to the wise, but always question. Truth and love are simple and ever present.

We need not seek initiations and intermediaries. We need only the awakening that allows us to see. Awakening comes uninvited from a flower, a person, a word of love, a crisis, or the wind on the water. This awakening may not even require a big experience, or a mysterious inner light. Inner visionary experiences can be overwhelmingly beautiful, but they are no more so than the outer visions we see each day in the universe. We have just become used to, numb to, the miracles in which we are living.

Meditation and spirituality come into being in the twinkling of an eye in any moment that allows us to pierce the veil of the ordinary, the repetitive, the dull. We need only the sensitivity of understanding and awareness—insight that reveals that we are already immersed in the miraculous, the holy, the sacred. It is the earth, the trees, the wind. It is the rivers, the stars, and the cosmos—and each person. It is the miracle of life, of consciousness itself; it is the immeasurable. The beauty of nature, the body, the hand, the eye, and the existence of love are all facets of this miraculous jewel. The self is not a tiny spark in all these things—it is all of these things. It is the All, and the universe is its face. We are at once the infinite and the infinitesimal, the eternal and ephemeral. We stand on the shoulders of the past seeing farther than ever before. We are the self-reflecting part viewing the whole, the observer and the observed, time-bound and timeless, our lives the prayer. Tat Twam Asi, *you are that!*

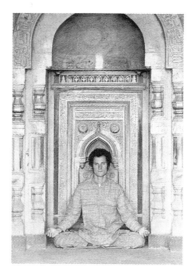

Ganga in Fatehpur Sikri, India. 1971.

# ABOUT THE AUTHOR—
## A Short Biography

Ganga White is a lifelong adventurer, explorer, and student of yoga. His odyssey began when he was eleven years old and saw the word "yogi" chalked on a school sidewalk. It being the late fifties, no doubt it was some baseball fan's favorite-player graffiti, but for Ganga, it seemed something foreign and the strangeness in it needed deciphering. He asked a kid on the playground, "What's a yogi?" and was told that yogis were "these guys in the Himalayas who could wave their hands and make a flower appear." In that instant he resolved to go there someday.

This vignette illustrates the offbeat leanings of Ganga's mind and the strength of his curiosity, even from an early age. The image of a yogi making flowers appear never left him. Always fascinated by nature, science, and electronics, he earned his amateur radio operator's license at age fourteen and spoke with people around the world on ham radio. He raced hot rods and earned his California State University tuition by fixing TVs and managing an electronics store. In 1966 he and a friend read *Black Like Me* and Errol Flynn's autobiography and decided to drop out and explore life, the civil rights movement, and the turbulent sixties. They traveled the country hitchhiking and hopping freight trains, eventually landing back on Sunset Strip in the heyday of the counterculture and participating in and conducting visionquests using the *Tibetan Book of the Dead*.

Ganga began his study in 1966 of yoga and comparative religion with the scholar Dr. Framroze Bode, a Zoroastrian high priest and Doctor of Religion in Los Angeles. Within a year he was living at the Sivananda Yoga Ashram in Canada, fixing their electronics and sound systems and meeting yogis and swamis from around the world. After a couple of years he mastered the most advanced asanas and practices. In 1967 he founded the Center for Yoga in Los Angeles and served as principle teacher for twenty-five years. He was credited with helping spearhead the new wave of yoga in America and hosted a continuous stream of yogis and masters, many on their first visits to Los Angeles, making their way to the U.S. and Canada. The list of luminaries includes Vishnudevananda, Venkatesa, Chidananda, Muktananda, Satchidananda, Pir Vilayat Khan, Ram Dass, Kalu Rimpoche, Allen Ginsberg, BKS Iyengar, and K. Pattabhi Jois.

Along the way Ganga founded yoga centers in major U.S. cities and served for five years as vice-president of the International Sivananda Yoga Vedanta Centers. He was designated the successor to Swami Vishnu, but left in 1973 due to philosophical differences so he could pursue and begin developing a non-dogmatic, contemporary vision of yoga. Throughout the late sixties and seventies, he traveled around the U.S. and the world, teaching and lecturing at universities and institutes and appearing on numerous television programs. Ganga has taught yoga to stars and celebrities, consulted on movie sets and television specials, and traveled with yogis and swamis in the U.S., Europe, and India. He organized and led yoga tours and pilgrimages to India, assisted in and conducted the first yoga teacher trainings in North America, and organized the first American fire walk with sacred firewalkers from South India, walking on hot coals himself in 1970. He participated in peace gatherings and flew in the Peter Max-painted peace plane dropping leaflets over the San Francisco war moratorium gathering in Golden Gate Park. He has been called one of the "architects of American yoga" and a "pioneer of yoga" by the *Yoga Journal.*

Always characterized by an inquiring mind, Ganga worked with polygraph expert Cleve Backster on plant responses in New York and with the Findhorn Community in Scotland in 1974, and in the mid-seventies to early eighties he studied with J. Krishnamurti in California, Switzerland, England, and India. In the early eighties he trained in homeopathy at Sivananda Homeo Clinic in the Himalayas and studied with BKS Iyengar in India and Ashtanga yoga with K. Pattabhi Jois.

In 1991, Ganga participated in the first international conference on Ayahuasca and medicinal plants in Brazil. He invited the leaders and shamans back to the U.S. to continue exploring these healing traditions and comparing them to the practices and teachings of yoga. Ganga was an invited delegate to the Wisdom Keepers Gathering at the Earth Summit in Brazil, journeyed in the Amazon region, and hosted a series of meetings with elders and scientists researching entheogens.

While Ganga has had extensive classical training in several prominent lineages of yoga, in Sanskrit, and yoga philosophy—he received the teaching title *Yoga Acharya* three times from the Sivananda Ashram, the Yoga Vedanta Forest University, Rishikesh, Himalayas, and the Yoga Niketan in India—he has always been an innovating and startlingly original yogi. He created partner yoga, and in 1981 Viking Penguin published his beautifully illustrated *Double Yoga,* still the definitive volume on this unique system for partner practice. Also during the seventies, Ganga was one of the early developers of Flow Yoga and introduced it at centers all over the country. Flow is now one of the most popular systems of yoga practice.

The first-ever yoga workout video, *The Flow Series,* was released in 1990 in collaboration with Tracey Rich, Ganga's wife and fellow teacher of more than twenty-four years. Their second video, *Total Yoga,* published by Gaiam/Living Arts in 1994, has sold more than 1.4 million copies and has set records as the number one yoga video in the U.S. and worldwide, and fourth best selling exercise video. In 2002 TimeWarner published a three-volume video series, *Total Yoga, The Flow Series—Earth, Water, Fire.*

In 1983 Ganga and Tracey founded the White Lotus Retreat in the hills of Santa Barbara, which the couple has directed ever since. To these forty acres in the coastal mountains, thousands of students from around the world have come for yoga workshops, continuing education, and advanced studies. Highly respected in yoga circles, the White Lotus Foundation and its beautifully rustic hillside retreat is a premier institute for yoga and teacher training in the U.S.

Students and colleagues have long appreciated Ganga as an inspiring and insightful instructor. He's able to communicate yoga's complex teachings and intricate dynamics, relating to others through his use of anecdotal experience, his down-to-earth way with language, and a wonderful sense of humor. Though Ganga has been bestowed—from Swami Venkatesananda—with the rare, honorific title *Yogiraj* and has a Sanskrit name, he is an iconoclast in the truest sense, a critical and free thinker who always questions traditional and ritualized beliefs, dogmatic systems, and authority of all kinds. His revolutionary teaching empowers the individual while retaining the essential truths of yoga.

A chalked sidewalk epiphany is a rare beginning for a world-renowned career, but within that young boy's need to know was a pattern of intellectual and experiential curiosity that has formed Ganga White and his unique perspective on life and the physical and spiritual discipline that is yoga.

—Evelyn de Buhr
8/15/2006

With Swami Vishnudevananda at the opening of Ganga's first yoga center. Los Angeles, 1967.

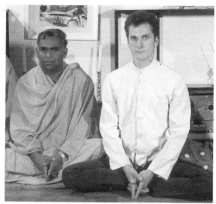

Don Josephson

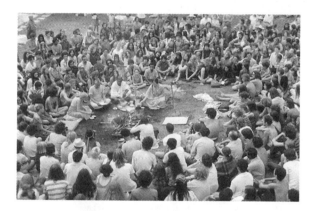

Firewalking ceremony with village priests from India. Val Morin, Canada, 1970.

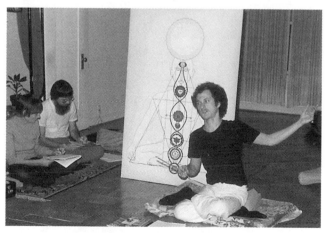

Leading the U.S.'s first yoga teacher training. Los Angeles, 1969.

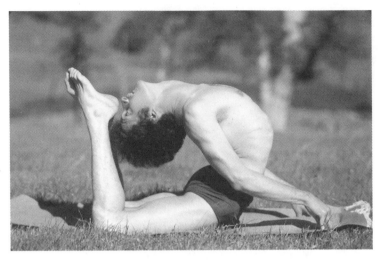

King Cobra Pose. Grass Valley, California, 1971.

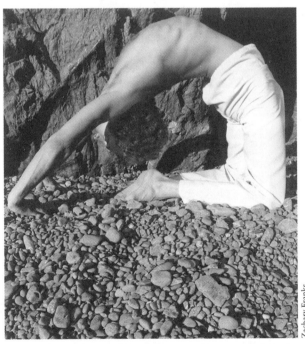

Zachary Franks

Diamond Pose. Mendocino, California, 1977.

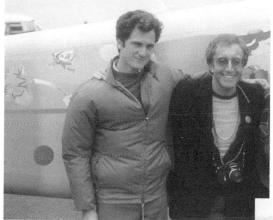

Teaching on tour with
Peter Sellers and the
Peter Max Peace Plane.
Ireland, 1971.

Swami Venkatesananda. Grass
Valley, California, 1972.

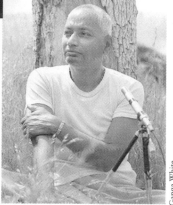

Ganga White

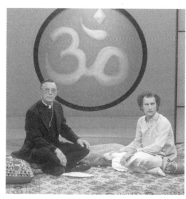

CBS special series on Eastern
religion. 1977.

Private demonstration for
Mohammed Ali (Full Bow Pose).
Miami, 1970.

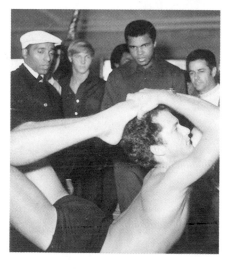

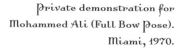

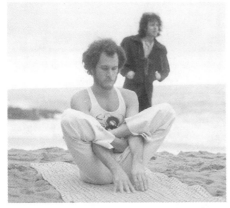

Filming *Aliens on Planet Earth* with musician Donovan. Malibu, California, 1976.

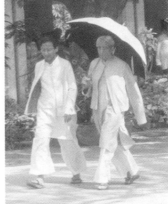

Touring with J. Krishnamurti. Rishi Valley, India, 1980.

Ganga White

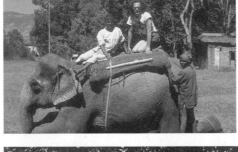

India jungle tour. Mudumulai, India, 1980.

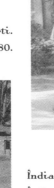

Sitting meditation. Mendocino, California, 1977.

Zachary Franks

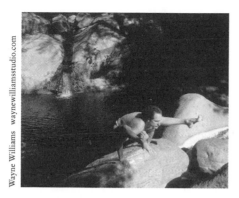

Wayne Williams   waynewilliamsstudio.com

Flying İnsect Pose. White Lotus retreat, Santa Barbara, California, 1990.

Cover photo of Ganga and Tracey for *Healing Lifestyles and Spas Magazine* (Stacked Lotus Pose). 2000.

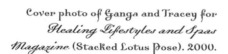

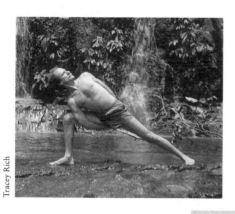

Tracey Rich

Charles Montague

Amazon jungle shamanic journey (Arm Locked Extended Warrior). 1993.

Tracey and Ganga assist Sting teaching his first yoga class. Los Angeles, 2003.

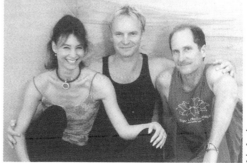

Jake Jacobson

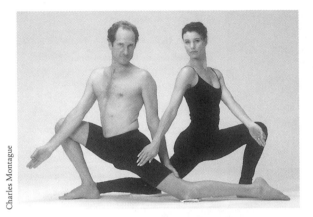

Charles Montague

Double Lunge Pose
with Tracey. White
Lotus retreat, Santa
Barbara, California,
2000.

Leg Head Tiptoe
Balance Pose.
Kennebunkport,
Maine, 1987.

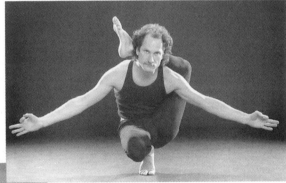

Ed Holcomb

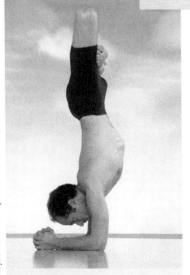

Wayne Williams   waynewilliamsstudio.com

Lotus Forearm Balance Pose.
Los Angeles, 2004.

# NOTES

1. There are thousands of translations of this important text, and Swami Venkates wrote one of his own: Swami Venkatesananda, *Enlightened Living: A New Interpretive Translation of The Yoga Sutras of Patanjali*, Sebastopol, Calif., Anahata Press, 1975.

2. J. Krishnamurti, *Freedom from the Known*, San Francisco, Harper, 1969, p. 15.

3. Pose? Posture? The words are interchangeable. Pose is more common, perhaps, but they mean the same thing.

4. Arthur Avalon, *The Serpent Power*, Madras, India, Ganesh and Co., 1924, and reprinted in 1974 by Dover Publications; also by Avalon, *Sakti and Sakta*, Madras, India, Ganesh and Co., 1918, reprinted in 2001 by Nesma Books India.

5. David Gordon White, *The Alchemical Body*, Chicago, University of Chicago Press, 1996; also by White, *The Kiss of the Yogini*, Chicago, University of Chicago Press, 2003.

6. *Siddhartha*, reprinted in 1981 by Bantam Classics.

7. Swami Venkatesananda, *The Concise Yoga Vasistha*, New York, State University of New York, 1984, a translation of the ancient text.

# INDEX

## A

Active holding, 119–21
Aging, 193–94
Ajna, 157
Alchemy, 83
Alignment, 69–71, 91–95
Amrita, 187–88
Anahata, 157
Arjuna, 64
Asanas. *See also* Practice
    active holding of, 119–21
    aligning and adjusting, 91–95
    classes of, 126–32
    long holding of, 121
    number of, 29, 45
    passive holding of, 120–21
    power of, 70
    sequencing of, 70
    as standing waves, 88
    tension and, 54–55
    as tools, 43–45
Ashtanga yoga, 16
Astral body, 153, 156, 159
Astronomical meditation, 190–92
Attention, 64
Avalon, Sir Arthur, 154
Ayahuasca, 188

## B

Backbends, 128–30
Balance, nature of, 108–9
Balancing poses, 128
Balancing Warrior, 34
Bandhas, 103–5
Beginner's mind, 7, 41
*Bhagavad Gita*, 20, 163
Bhakti yoga, 18–19, 21
Body
    feedback from, 46–48, 92
    meditation, 183

    -mind systems, 27, 30–35
    types, 59–60
Brahma, 28
Brahmacharya, 5
Breath
    central role of, 32, 100
    meditation, 180
    pranayama, 32, 99–103
    ujjayi, 66–67
    using, 65–66
Buddha, 200

## C

Candle meditation, 180–81
Car yoga, 122–23
Chakras
    color and, 154, 158
    daily life and, 164–66
    as energy centers, 156–59
    etymology of, 156
    history of, 153–54
    levels of being and, 159–62
    number of, 153–54
    relationship of, to science, 155–56
Circulatory system, 31–32
Competition, 58–59
Concentration, 64, 176
Consciousness
    origin of, 154–55
    self-, 142
Control, 17–18, 97
Cooling, 50–52
Corpse pose, 74, 91
Cosmic polarity, 162–64

## D

Death
    meditation, 192–93
    mystery of, 211–14
Denial, 17

Devotion, 18–19, 19–20
Digestive system, 32–33
Discipline, 62–63
Diversity, loss of, 201–2
Doubt, 19
Downward Dog, 31, 131–32
Dynamic holding, 119–21

E
Edges, surfing, 95–97
Einstein, Albert, 162
Eliminative system, 32–33
Emotions, 35
Endocrine system, 33–34
Energy
    body, 84–86
    chakras and, 156–59
    cosmic polarity and, 162–64
    life as dance of, 84
    lines of, 88–90
    mental, 91
    standing waves of, 87, 88
    upward and downward, 86–87
    withdrawing, 90–91
Enlightenment, 208–11
Extended Warrior, 93

F
Faith, 19
Fear, 57–58
Feedback, 46–48, 92
Fire, 180–81
Flexibility, 48–50, 68, 95–96
Flow yoga, 114–15
Forward bends, 130–31

G
Gaia, 164
Goals, 43–45
God, oneness with, 17, 18, 19, 200–201
Gorakhnath, 28
Gravity, 86–87
Grounding, 160
Group practice, 76
Gunas, 71

H
Half Moon, 34
Hamsa-ji, 44–45
Hamstrings, 124–26
Handstand, 57, 131–32
Hatha yoga. See also Practice
    as art and science, 26
    benefits of, 25–26, 30
    body-mind systems in, 27, 30–35
    control and surrender in, 97–99
    etymology of, 25, 26, 49
    origins of, 16–17, 28–30
    polarity in, 26, 53
    popularity of, 25
    Raja yoga and, 16, 97
Headstand, 31, 57, 131–32
Healing resonance, 145
Heating, 50–52
Heisenberg, Werner, 163
Herbs, 187–89
Hesse, Herman, 186
Holograms, 155–56

I
Iccha, 72
Ida, 156
Injuries. See also Pain
    causes of, 135, 146–48
    local intelligence and, 141–45
    old, 147–48
    preventing, 135–37, 146–48
    sympathetic resonance and, 145–46
    working with, 148–50
Intelligence
    of the body, 46–48
    definition of, 8
    local, 141–45
    of plants, 188
Interconnectedness, 210
Intuitive Flow yoga, 116–18
Inversions, 131–32
Isometric pressure, 106
Isotonic pressure, 106
Iyengar, B.K.S., 144

# J

Jalandhara Bandha, 104, 105
Jnana, 72
Jnana yoga, 19–20, 21

# K

Karma, 213–14
Karma yoga, 20–21
Knowledge, 7–8, 10
Koans, 10–11
Kramer, Joel, 89, 95
Krishnamurti, J., 6, 163
Kriya, 72
Kundalini
    awakening, 158
    sacrum and, 157
    Shakti, 157

# L

Laghima, 75
Leverage, 105–7
Life
    as dance of energy, 84
    death and, 192–93, 211–14
    as meditation, 169, 171–72, 195
    navigating, 214–16
Light, 163, 210
Local intelligence, 141–45
Locks, 103–5
Long holding, 121
Lotus pose, 79
Love, 10, 17
Lumbar, 123–24

# M

Mahavakyas, 9
Manipura, 157
Mantra meditation, 182
Matsyendranath, 28, 29
Meditation
    on aging, 193–94
    approaches to, 170–71
    astronomical or science, 190–92
    body, 183
    breath, 180
    candle, 180–81

concentration and, 176
death, 192–93
definition of, 169–71
goals of, 171, 172–73
life as, 169, 171–72, 195
mantra, 182
nature and, 184–87
reasons for, 171
relationship and, 184
sacred plants and, 187–89
self-study, 183
sitting, 176–79
solitude and, 183–84
sound and music in, 181–82
techniques for, 174–94
Mental-emotional systems, 35
Mental energy, 91
Meridians, 156
Milky Way galaxy, 190–91
Mind
    beginner's, 7, 41
    capacities of, 172–73
    control systems, 170, 182
    emotions and, 35
    interrelationships of body and,
        27, 30–35
    practice and, 56–57
Mula Bandha, 87, 103, 104, 105
Muladhara, 157
Muscular system, 31, 69
Music, 181–82

# N

Nadis, 156
Narada, 212–13
Nature, spirituality of, 184–87
Neck, 123–24
Nervous system, 34–35
Neti Neti, 10

# O

OM, 181, 182
Oneness
    experience of, 18, 19, 190, 200–201
    loss of diversity and, 201–2

**P**

Pain. *See also* Injuries
   function of, 137–38, 140
   relieving, 141–42
   types of, 140–41, 143
Paracelsus, 188
Parsvakonasana, 93
Paschimottanasana, 120
Passive holding, 120–21
Patanjali, 3, 4–5, 16, 100, 173–74
Perfection, 61–62
Pingala, 157
Plants, sacred, 187–89
Practice. *See also* Asanas; Hatha yoga;
Meditation; Yoga
   aggressive, 147
   alignment and, 69–71
   asanas as tools in, 43–45
   attention and, 64
   body types and, 59–60
   breathing and, 65–67
   competition and comparison in,
     58–59
   concentration and, 64
   dedicating time for, 40–41
   discipline and, 62–63
   enjoying, 80
   fear and, 57–58
   feedback and, 46–48, 92
   flow and grace in, 74–75
   goals in, 43–45, 61–62
   group, 76
   heating and cooling in, 50–52
   inner- and outer-directed, 55–56,
     115
   integrating, into daily life, 77–80,
     122–23
   lifelong, 39–40
   limitations on, 56–58
   long view of, 42–43
   odd-day, 122
   perfection and, 61–62
   personal, 75–77
   presence and, 39–41
   regularity of, 62–63, 147
   relaxation and, 73–74

   rhythms and seasons of, 53–54
   spine and, 68–69
   strength and flexibility in, 48–50
   structural integrity and, 70, 118–19
   surfing the edges in, 95–97
   symmetry and, 69–71, 122
   taking time off from, 63, 74
   tension and, 54–55
   three qualities and, 71–72
   three root principles and, 72
   traction, torque, and leverage in,
     105–7
Prana, 35, 99–100, 101
Pranayama, 32, 99–103
Pranic energy system, 35
Presence, 39–41
Psoas, 124–26

**Q**

Quadriceps, 124–26
Questioning, 10, 19–20

**R**

Rajas, 71–72
Raja yoga, 16, 17–18, 21, 97
Receptivity, 9
Reincarnation, 213–14
Relationship, 184
Relaxation, 73–74
Respiratory system, 32
RICES, 148–49
Rituals, 206–7

**S**

Sahasrara, 157
Santosha, 208
Sattwa, 71–72
Savasana, 74, 91
Science meditation, 190–92
Seated Boat, 34
Seated Forward Fold, 120
Self-centeredness, 21
Self-consciousness, 142
Self-image, 57
Self-study, 183
Serpent imagery, 157

Sexuality, 17
Shakti, 29, 161, 163
Shoulderstand, 31, 34, 79, 124, 131–32
Siddhartha, 186
Sitting, 78–79
Siva, 28–29, 75, 161, 163
Skeletal system, 30–31, 69
Snake imagery, 157
Solitude, 183–84
Soma, 187–89
Spinal twists, 65, 131, 143–44
Spine
    cervical, 123–24
    compression of, 68
    lumbar, 123–24
    toning, 68–69
Spirituality
    approaches to, 203
    changing and growing, 202–8
    of nature, 184–87
    organization and, 206
    tradition and, 199, 204
Spiritual materialism, 204–5
Standing poses, 127
Standing waves, 87, 88
Stars, gazing at, 190–92
Strength, 48–50, 96
Structural archetypes, 119
Structural integrity, 70, 118–19
Subtle body, 153, 156, 159
Sun Salutation, 50, 65, 127
Sushumna, 157
Svadishhtana, 157
Swadhyaya, 183
Sweating, 51–52
Symmetry, 69–71, 122
Sympathetic resonance, 145–46

T
Tamas, 71–72
Tantra yoga, 16–17
Tao Te Ching, 9
Tat Twam Asi, 9–10, 19

Tension, 73
Time, mystery of, 212–13
Torque, 105–7
Traction, 105–7
Tradition, 3, 4–7, 11, 204
Transformation, 28
Tratakum, 180–81
Tree pose, 108
Triangle pose, 84

U
Uddiyana Bandha, 104, 105
Ujjayi breath, 66–67
Uncertainty Principle, 163

V
Vedanta, 10
Venkates, Swami, 3, 5, 104
Vichara, 194
Vishnu, 28, 212–13
Vishuddha, 157
Vivekananda, Swami, 16

W
Warm-ups, 50–51
White, David Gordon, 154

Y
Yama, 100
Yoga. See also Hatha yoga; Practice
    advancing in, 109
    balance and, 108–9
    body types and, 59–60
    etymology of, 15
    integrating, into daily life, 77–80, 122–23
    interpretations of, 3, 4–7, 15
    tradition and, 3, 4–7, 11, 28
    types of, 15–21, 26
    in the West, 3
    wholeness of, 21–22
The Yoga Sutras of Patanjali, 3
The Yoga Vasistha, 212

For more information about Ganga White,
his workshops, books, videos, and DVDS, visit:

**The White Lotus Foundation**
Santa Barbara, California
(805) 964-1944
*www.whitelotus.org*
*info@whitelotus.org*